Arthritis Reversed

Second Edition

Arthritis Reversed

Groundbreaking 30-Day
Arthritis Relief Action Plan

Dr. Mark Wiley

Join the Tens of Thousands Who Use This Groundbreaking, Natural Approach to Prevent, Slow, and Reduce the Painful Symptoms of Arthritis . . . Today!

Disclaimer

The information in this book is provided for informational purposes only and is not a substitute for professional medical advice. The author and publisher make no legal claims, express or implied, and the material is not intended to replace the services of a physician.

The author, publisher and/or copyright holder assume no responsibility for the loss or damage caused, or allegedly caused, directly or indirectly by the use of information contained in this book. The author and publisher specifically disclaim any liability incurred from the use or application of the contents of this book.

Throughout this book trademarked names are referenced. Rather than putting a trademark symbol in every occurrence of a trademarked name, we state that we are using the names in an editorial fashion only and to the benefit of the trademark owner with no intention of infringement of the trademark.

ISBN: 978-0-615-97650-1
First Edition, 2013
Second Edition, 2014

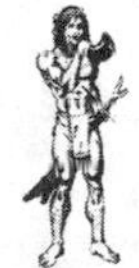

Tambuli Media
Spring House, PA
www.TambuliMedia.com

Praise for "Arthritis Reversed"

"Dr. Mark is one of the great health and wellness minds of our generation."

– Herb Borkland, MA
Emmy-Award Winning Broadcaster

"Dr. Mark Wiley is one of the most knowledgeable health and wellness experts I know. I'm certain you'll find this book to be an invaluable resource."

– Jesse Cannone, CFT, CPRS
The Healthy Back Institute

"Dr. Wiley is one of the most clear thinkers and writers in complimentary medicine today. This book is revolutionary and yet it is so simple to follow each step of his plan. Arthritis and the fear and stigma of arthritis causes many people to unnecessarily accept a lower quality of life. Armed with Dr. Wiley's excellent book, I hope thousands of people will take back control of their lives, follow his plan and live the life they were born to enjoy."

– Dr. Glenn P. Lobo, DO, LicAc, MBAcC
The Caring Osteopath

"Dr. Mark Wiley's approach is both personal and practical. Since he 'knows what it is like' to experience arthritis."

– Dr. Brett D. Cardonick, DC
Cardonick Chiropractic PC

"'Arthritis Reversed' is an ode to pain and discomfort. It is a road map to recovery for a very complex far reaching disease: arthritis. More than that, it is a skilled and learned man's work at deciphering the human body and a management program, all rolled into one. Dr. Mark Wiley took all the scientific research, the traditional holistic approaches and his own personal experience and has now supplied the public with simple answers to a painful condition. This truly is a book to own and use. 'Arthritis Reversed' is a road map to recovery from arthritic pain and will help you get your life back."

– Dr. Robert del Medico, DAc, CertOT, CHt, RMT
Gestus Manuel Therapy, Advance Family Chiropractic

"Dr. Mark Wiley has written an incredibly informative book that can help everyday people deal with and reverse the effects of arthritis, utilizing natural methods with no side effects. Dr. Wiley is to be commended for taking decades worth of research on natural wellness practices and creating an integrated approach to optimal health and well-being. I wholeheartedly recommend this and any other book by Dr. Wiley to anyone who is suffering from Arthritis or other health issues. Do not let arthritis rule your life! Get this book and see what it can do for you. It has helped my patients gain more control over their lives."

– Dr. Dale Dugas, DOM DiplOM LicAc
Dugas Acupuncture and Chinese Herbal Medicine

"If you have arthritis, you need to read this book. Dr. Mark Wiley is a learned healer with a mind for truth about pain and how to relieve it."

– Alan Orr, LAc
The Chinese Medicine Academy

"Our readers have asked for the perfect resource to help them overcome arthritis pain. We've shared invaluable bits of wisdom from Dr. Wiley with them whenever we can. With the release of *Arthritis Reversed,* he's drawn back the curtain and given the world the definitive Arthritis Relief Action Plan so everyone can live pain free."

– Steve Coombes
Managing Editor, Live Pain Free

This book is for YOU – the arthritis sufferer – who is tired of letting pain control your life. In these pages, you will find the keys to lasting relief.

CONTENTS

Foreword by Dr. Robert Chu

I am pleased to write this forward for my good friend and fellow researcher and clinician, Dr. Mark Wiley. His work here will give anyone suffering from pain and arthritis a host of new ways to control their pain, and to consider other options, rather than using over-the-counter medications and/or conventional medicine.

He exposes the myths of arthritis, various types of arthritis and risks, and the issues that mainstream medicine can actually exacerbate. Dr. Wiley explains the biggest mistakes made in treating arthritis, and the inflammatory response and how to curtail that with foods, control of emotions, reducing stress, and natural supplements that can empower you to relieve your pain.

Finally, Dr. Wiley empowers you with a complete month-long plan to reduce your inflammation, set goals to curtail the pain, and put into action all you need to master arthritis relief. I highly recommend this book to anyone suffering from any form of arthritis.

– Robert Chu, PhD, L.Ac, QME
International Lecturer on Acupuncture and Chinese Medicine
Clinical Supervisor, Emperor's College of Traditional Oriental Medicine
DAOM lecturer, Disney Family Cancer Center

A Personal Message from Dr. Mark Wiley

Hello, I'm Dr. Mark Wiley and I've spent decades researching and mastering natural wellness practices around the world. I've taken those techniques and pioneered a powerful integrated mind/body approach to optimal health and well-being. It's a self-directed (do-it-yourself, DIY) kind of approach. And it is based on this fundamental truth:

You don't have to live in pain. You don't have to suffer a chronic health condition. The arthritic pain and inflammation you "deal with" every day do not need to be permanent fixtures in your life. I will tell you why and show you how to overcome them.

I know you wish it were true … and I am here to tell you, it is!

Yet, from early on, you are taught to "manage" and "mask the symptoms of" and "live with" your poor health conditions. This is perverse. It goes against our homeostatic (self-balancing) nature. What's more, despite lackluster results, too many people keep following the practices of a healthcare system that simply has not delivered on its promises.

Are we doing this because we don't realize it's not working? Surely, our chronic daily pain and suffering is the indication it's not working.

Simply put, mainstream medicine fails to eradicate our everyday pains, illnesses and diseases. It fails because it is *passive* and *reactionary* and thus unable to prevent you from experiencing chronic health conditions like heart disease, diabetes, hypertension, obesity, stress, anxiety, depression, headache, back pain, tendonitis and hundreds of others … including arthritis.

And this model will always fall short because it uses *disease* as its basis of finding *health*. That is, you see your primary care physician when you are ill, the doctor diagnoses your illness, labels the disease, then prescribes a protocol for treating that disease or symptoms. Your personal health issues are "managed" by prescription medication, various therapies and surgery. Natural treatment can also fall into this category, if the approach is relief of symptoms and not correction on underlying (root) causes. While treating symptoms of pain and inflammation are necessary for immediate relief, it must be done as an intermediary step while implementing a truly corrective approach, such as the one presented in this book. After all, any model based simply on symptomatic relief (whether modern or traditional) can never hope to resolve your daily wellness problems.

The important thing, as a person suffering with arthritis, is to see and know that the solution to your daily suffering is grounded in a five-part process called the Arthritis Relief Action Plan:

Arthritis Relief Action Plan

Part 1: Educate yourself about the real causes and solutions of arthritis

Part 2: Reduce the current level of symptoms you are experiencing

Part 3: Halt or significantly reduce the worsening of your arthritic condition

Part 4: Prevent the symptoms from flaring to improve your quality of life

Part 5: Regenerate healthy tissue to reverse the damage done

These five parts can be achieved. In fact, for the best and fastest results, you should work toward them at the same time. One does not come before the other, with the exception of educating yourself as to what to do and how to do it. I have written this book with the express purpose of delivering to you, in one place, all of the information you need to satisfy all five parts of the arthritis equation.

When it comes to arthritis relief, I am sure you have spoken to many specialists. So why should you believe in what I say? Well, for starters, I know how you feel. Like you, as I went from doctor to doctor, desperately hoping for relief, no one could help me. Every day was a soul-destroying battle with neck and shoulder pain, mid-back pain, hip pain and head pain. Pain, pain, pain.

You see, I suffered from severe chronic headaches and musculoskeletal pain my entire life. While I was trying to sleep one night about nine months ago, from seemingly out of nowhere my hip started pounding, throbbing in pain. The pain radiated down the front of my leg and under my knee. It was very painful and I went to get X-rays and an MRI to see what was wrong.

As it turns out, now in my middle age, I have been diagnosed with arthritis of the left hip. This was no fault of my own. My arthritis is secondary to a slipped capital femoral epiphysis. That is just a fancy way of saying when I was around 10 or 12, the head of my thighbone slipped slightly off its growth plate. This caused the ball-end of the thighbone to connect off center with the socket joint of the hip. This caused chronic pain, muscle contraction, limited range of motion and, over the past three decades, osteoarthritis. As a result, I have been advised by orthopedic surgeons to have my left hip replaced. No thank you.

Unlike some chronic pain sufferers, I was fortunate enough to have familial support. My parents are both healthcare professionals. Unfortunately, even with their love, direction and referral to experts in various specialty fields, the suffering was constant, unbearable and unrelenting. I was forever putting myself in front of medical doctors, osteopaths, naturopaths, chiropractors, physical therapists, psychologists, allergists, body workers, hypnotists and dietitians. No treatment or surgery had lasting results.

I became proactive in college. In addition to studying medical anthropology, I was in close contact with dozens of mind/body health practitioners around the country. I became a research assistant at Harvard Medical School, looking into how to combine various mind/body methods for pain relief and even using martial art drills as vehicles to create altered states of consciousness. Yet despite all this, the net results were underwhelming. I was finally forced to face the fact that conventional Western medicine and many of the so-called "complementary medicines" were unable to heal me. So I became the Marco Polo of pain.

I began traveling, tracking down rumors of cures for pain and suffering to be found in far-away places with strange-sounding names. Reiki and QiGong in Japan, tui na in Taiwan, acupuncture and traditional herbs in Singapore, faith healing and bone-setting in the Philippines, spiritualists and medicine men in Malaysia. Been there, done that, designed the T-shirt. Yes, as with Western doctoring there was some short-term relief, but the pain always returned. Always. Then one day, I had had enough and decided to make a final desperate change in my life's direction.

What did I do?

I went back to school, thinking that if I had the necessary background in human anatomy and physiology that I could better understand and assimilate the methods of the great healing traditions. And I was right! I earned a Master's Degree in Health Care Management also earned doctorates in Acupuncture and Oriental Medicine (OMD) and Alternative Medicine (PhD). Over the past 15 years of treating patients, lecturing worldwide and writing books and hundreds of articles, I developed a proactive self-directed, self-cure model of optimal health and pain-free living. The invaluable information found in this book is derived from the principles of that method. The solutions for each specific disease or condition – like arthritis – is set into the plan template, for specificity.

The Arthritis Relief Action Plan entails some key lifestyle changes. These are necessary when it comes to defeating the debilitating symptoms of arthritis. While lifestyle changes are the only way to correct imbalances and *remain in an optimal state of health, they are not always difficult.* Sure, some may be more difficult than others for some people, depending on their habits. But some of the suggested changes are very simple and even fun.

With this in mind, "Arthritis Reversed" is divided into three sections, and each should be read in sequence for best results.

Section One: The Many Causes, Myths and Triggers of Arthritis aims to educate you on the what's, why's and how's of arthritis in easily understandable language, less jargon and more explanation. By understanding the arthritis situation from many perspectives (not just medical, but holistic and alternative, too), you will see the condition for what it really is. This section lays out *the obvious and the hidden causes of arthritis* and the many things that make it worse – many of which, as you will learn, you have direct control over.

Section Two: Natural Solutions Your Doctor Doesn't Know provides an overview of the most powerful and accessible treatment options for arthritis. It discusses both Eastern and Western methods, from bodywork to energy medicine to pain creams, diet and supplementation. It offers a broad view on the many options available to you for relief, some of which you may not have been aware of. It aims to give you insights into each so you can find one or several that may work best for you.

Section Three: The 30-Day Arthritis Relief Action Plan is set into three "30-Day Action Plans" that pull all of this information together for you. It gives you the "how to do it" approach, by putting into place a series of steps, and an action plan, that you can manage over a brief period to help you achieve the five-part solution mentioned above. Its only aim is to provide you with a map that will lead you to arthritis relief and, ultimately, a better quality of life.

I would like to point out how important it is to have a mentor when dealing with health and wellness. It is difficult to do on your own, even with the Internet offering scads of articles at your fingertips. Sure, a day spent surfing the Net could turn up hundreds of separate articles that discuss some of the things found in this book. But is that enough? I don't think so. Without a context in which to understand and place the information, how can you hope to implement it in an appropriate and significant way? I have the education and experience necessary to assimilate the individual parts of the arthritis puzzle and then present the parts as a cohesive whole. So let me be your mentor, let this book provide you with the proper context in which to understand arthritis, its symptoms and the methods available to overcome its debilitating effects on your life.

In the pages of this book, I show you how to determine the underlying – and sometimes hidden – causes of your arthritic symptoms. These are actually obvious root causes and contributors that are only "hidden" because you have not (yet) been taught to look for and identify them. I'll show you how to do this and then how to use that knowledge to reduce your pain and halt or slow the progression of the condition, typically within 30 to 90 days. The information and plan is comprehensive, easy to understand and set out in a way that you can follow. And don't worry: what you'll discover in the following pages will pass your "common sense" test with flying colors. As you read, you'll find yourself nodding along and telling yourself, "Yes, this makes sense." The information and program in this book worked for me and it can work for you, too. Let's get started on overcoming your arthritis so you, too, can live a pain-free life.

– Dr. Mark Wiley

SECTION 1:

The Many Causes, Myths and Triggers of Arthritis

CHAPTER 1

The Eight Biggest Arthritis Myths

For any wellness action plan to work there must be a clear understanding of the various aspects involved. The puzzle pieces must be identified before steps can be taken to piece them together. This all begins with clearing up the myths and setting forth the facts of the situation, and this chapter aims to do that for arthritis.

The line between fact and fiction is often thin. People form their beliefs on what they think sounds *reasonable* based on their education on a given topic, whether they gain that information from a friend or doctor, read it in a magazine or online, or saw and heard it on the news. Myths in healthcare take shape (and indeed take on a life of their own) when a sound bite or piece of information is spread and made public as fact before the person or companies releasing that information have the necessary *context* in which to consider the so-called facts. Without a context in which to understand something, any piece of content (information) is meaningless.

When it comes to diseases and conditions like arthritis, the pain and symptoms can wreak havoc on a life. If left unchecked, the quality of life of the one suffering arthritis can be destroyed, as well as the life of those close to them. As a person suffering from arthritis, you know how difficult it can be to maintain your quality of life, your daily routines, your cheery disposition and positive outlook regarding your disease and your life. This is especially true during times of extreme pain and immobility. Please know and believe me when I say, "severe pain, immobility and negative outlook do not have to be the center of your life." This book aims to help you believe otherwise.

To begin, I wish to present you with seven of the most common myths surrounding arthritis. Please take your time as you read this chapter and consider each myth. For those myths you believe, be open to understanding the myths and then believing the facts.

It is my sincere hope that by understanding these basic yet simple facts you will find a more positive view of your arthritic condition and, as a result, be more inclined to follow the therapeutic solutions found in later chapters. After all, a firm belief based in fact goes a long way toward beginning and maintaining a wellness program, especially when one is facing daily pain and physical and emotional debilitation. Let's look at those myths.

MYTH #1:
Rheumatoid Arthritis (RA) and Osteoarthritis (OA) are the Same

Perhaps the most pervasive myth of all is the notion that there is only one type of arthritis and it just happens to have different symptoms for different people. While it is easy to see how people might think that, it is not the case. In fact, there are over 100 different types of arthritis; the three most common being osteoarthritis (OA), rheumatoid arthritis (RA) and juvenile arthritis (JA).

While rheumatoid and juvenile arthritis are *diseases*– autoimmune diseases, to be precise – osteoarthritis (OA) is not a disease at all. It is a symptom of joint degeneration.

Autoimmune diseases, like rheumatoid and juvenile arthritis (and type I diabetes, lupus, multiple sclerosis, etc.), are progressive and associated with a systemic autoimmune disorder. That means the body makes antibodies that attack its own tissues and joints when triggered by some unknown event. Such triggers are known to include a reaction to a virus, the flu shot and stress. In the case of RA and JA, the joints are affected from the internal imbalance.

On the other hand, osteoarthritis is the result of any combination of several external factors, including traumatic physical injury and excessive sports or physical activities over the course of decades. This causes wear and tear of the joints, as well as of the cartilage separating the joints and the surrounding tissues (tendon and muscle).

Therefore, "arthritis" can be correctly thought of as a disorder of the joints with two main causes: (1) incorrect autoimmune response and (2) wear and tear on the joints. So while the symptoms may be similar, RA and JA are diseases while OA is a symptom of a structural joint problem brought on by external stressors.

Just having basic clarity on this first myth alone should provide you with some anxiety relief. After all, most people with arthritis have osteoarthritis (only one percent have RA). Simply knowing that it is not a disease and that its symptoms are quite manageable with natural, non-invasive approaches should provide you with enough hope for change that you find almost immediate improvement in your daily outlook.

MYTH #2:
Arthritis Is a Normal Part of Aging and Only Affects the Elderly

If you look around it is easy to see how this myth formed and took hold. There are plenty of elderly afflicted with arthritic conditions. And since many elderly can be seen with the visible signs of arthritis (i.e., misshapen hands, walkers and wheelchairs), one might conclude that arthritis is a normal part of the aging process. However, this is not the case anymore.

To begin correcting this myth it is important to know that rheumatoid and juvenile arthritis are autoimmune diseases and, therefore, have nothing to do with aging. Osteoarthritis, on the other hand, is a result of joint wear and tear based in injury and/or overuse, which can come on at any time – or not at all. As such, OA also is not a "normal" part of the aging process.

By keeping the immune system strong and stable, eating right, exercising right and taking care of bone and joint health, the onset and debilitating effects of arthritis need not be part of your aging process. And with better diagnosis and natural treatment remedies and therapies available, when you find you have the condition you can stop it and reduce or even reverse its symptoms, so they will not progress into your senior years.

MYTH #3:
If You Don't Look "Sick," You Don't Have Rheumatoid Arthritis

If one is only looking to the outward signs and symptoms of RA to know if they have it, they will be amiss. Even when people do not have the visible outward signs of rheumatoid arthritis, such as red swollen joints and misshapen fingers, they can still suffer symptoms, like joint pain, fatigue and a general sense of feeling unwell. Again, RA is an autoimmune disease and can be active before visible signs of it manifest.

The best way to know if you have, or are at risk for, RA is speak to your primary care physician, look into family history and do some blood work. Knowing your risks ahead of time, or early enough in the continuum of the disease, will help you get a jump on the symptoms and immune regulation needed to live a better quality of life.

MYTH #4:
If You Have Arthritis, You Should not Exercise

This is a myth most believed by those suffering the symptoms of arthritic pain and inflammation. Decades ago patients were told not to exercise because it would rub the joints and make things worse. This is incorrect. While it is true that depending on your arthritis type and conditions certain exercises should be avoided, this is not a blanket statement about all forms of exercise.

The fact is, a certain amount of exercise can greatly help reduce the symptoms of arthritis. Most often, those with arthritis in the hips and hands feel pain in the joints and inflammation and/or contraction in the muscles and tissues around those joints. However, part of what is contributing to the pain and stiffness is the limited range of motion within the joint structure that has happened as a result of not exercising.

The first step is to begin exercising slowly, lightly and with limits so as not to worsen or aggravate the conditions. Moving each joint slowly at first helps lubricate the joints and stretch the muscles. Strengthening exercises can help stabilize the arthritis joint structures. This in turn helps bring fresh blood, and thus oxygen and nutrients, to the area, which decreases inflammation, stiffness and pain. Exercise can increase in rigorousness and time as you are able.

The myth that one must rest and not exercise with arthritis no longer holds water. In fact, the National Institutes of Health (NIH) advocates exercises to help keep your muscles strong and your joints flexible … and to reduce the symptoms of depression, which can be common among people with a long-term illness like rheumatoid arthritis.

MYTH #5:
Different Climates Have No Effect on Arthritis

This myth is especially troublesome to me. To explain why, it is necessary to understand that there is truth within the myth, depending on the context of the conversation. According to the National Institutes of Health (NIH), there is no scientific evidence to support the notion that cold weather or environments cause arthritis or alter its course, or that warm weather can reverse or cure arthritis. All of this is true.

However, the important issue here is that both cold and warm weather can affect arthritis in negative or positive ways. Climate does play a role in how one experiences the symptoms of their arthritis. Cold weather constricts muscles, tendons and blood vessels, causing constriction around the joints, and thus pain and limited range of motion. Heat allows muscles to expand and blood to flow, and so relieves compression around joints and helps move fresh blood into the arthritis area. This reduces pain and stiffness and increases range of motion. Damp environments (whether warm or cold) cause inflammation around joints, and thus restrict movement and cause pain.

So while cold weather does not cause arthritis and warm weather does not cure it, it is clear that climate does play a role in how one experiences their arthritic condition and the symptoms involved therein. Therefore, temperature and climate should not be ignored when putting into place an arthritis relief action plan.

MYTH #6:
Arthritis Will Lead to Disability, Wheelchair and the Nursing Home

This myth is a hard one to bust, especially since it is formed and held in place by individual belief systems. As a result of our history of poor arthritis diagnosis, treatment and prevention methods, many who contracted arthritis did end up with a walker, in a wheelchair and living in assisted environments. Seeing them today can make one think the same will happen to you. However, what used to be fact is now fiction.

The first thing to understand is that arthritis is a continuum; it is not one size fits all. Moreover, as awareness of the RA disease and the OA condition increases, improved medical tests have become more specific to diagnose it sooner so treatment and preventive measures can be put into place. Three of the common blood tests are: measure the rheumatoid factor (RF), citrullinated peptide antibodies (anti-CCP), and erythrocyte sedimentation rate (ESR). Moreover, with information on diet, supplementation and with aided therapies like chiropractic, acupuncture, quantum touch and others, there are many restorative options available to halt its progression (if it is already there) and prevent it (if not).

Rheumatoid arthritis is the more difficult of the two most common types to control, as it is an autoimmune disease. But early detection and stabilization of the immune system can help keep it from progressing too rapidly. In fact, a study in the *Journal of Rheumatology* found that "after 10 years, 94 percent of the patients managed daily life activities independently."[1] This is promising indeed, especially since those in the study did not have a wide blanket of options at their disposal. Moreover, supplementation and change of diet and various therapies can reduce its symptoms while strengthening the affected and surrounding joint areas.

Osteoarthritis is easier to account for, stop and manage symptoms as they are mostly related to lifestyle and activity choices, bone and joint health and weight. Thus, the notion that if you get arthritis your history is written and you will end up in a wheelchair or in assisted living is no longer valid today. That is, if one takes the necessary steps, as detailed in this book.

MYTH #7:
Arthritis Sufferers Have To Live In Pain

This is a huge myth that is widely believed. Why? Because many arthritis sufferers *do* live in pain, with daily stiffness and inflammation. They are suffering greatly, yet needlessly. Why? Because they don't know all of the parts of the arthritis puzzle. Knowing them instills knowledge and knowledge provides the impetus and power for change.

By engaging in mind/body exercises to reduce stress, eating an anti-inflammatory diet, stretching, exercising, taking proper supplementation, using therapeutic creams and seeing practitioners for complementary wellness visits, you can greatly reduce, if not almost completely remove, the daily throbbing pain of arthritis. Inflammation decreases, blood flow increases, joint pressure reduces, joint support strengthens and pain slips away. While it takes time and effort, and a lifestyle change, you do not have to live your life in debilitating pain just because you have arthritis.

Will there be a certain level of pain associated with your arthritic condition, even after mindfully doing all of the steps and taking all of the advice in this book? Perhaps, but it should be nowhere near the levels you feel today. Even with the best treatment plan, the best healthcare providers, the best supplements and diet there are so many things to control. These include sleep patterns, stress levels, genetic makeup, and potential slips and falls that can increase your pain. However, you can control many of these, so you do have the means to reduce significantly the pain associated with arthritis.

MYTH #8:
Arthritis Can't Be Reversed

The notion that the damage done by arthritis cannot be reversed is perhaps the biggest myth of all. It is easy to see why people think this, and how the myth started, but it simply is untrue. You see, many of the "common beliefs" about arthritis are derived from a Western medical point of view. This view believes nothing can be done to reverse damage, and so patients need to manage their condition as best they can. In other words, symptomatic relief only. However, traditional and holistic medicines have natural methods for increasing bone density, rebuilding bone and regenerating soft tissue. In other words, a natural approach to reversing damage done by arthritis based on using supplements, topical creams and energy medicine. In the chapters that follow you will learn about these natural approaches and how they can help you.

Concluding Thoughts

It is my sincere wish that you not suffer the many debilitating symptoms of arthritis and that they not derail your life. I hope that you brought an open mind to my explanation of why the above seven myths do not hold water and understand that you are not prisoner to them. While it may be true that these eight myths are popularly believed, they are not grounded in irrefutable fact. Dismiss these myths and learn the facts of the situation so you can change your arthritis experience by, in many cases, preventing the progression of both rheumatoid and osteoarthritis. At the same time, you will reduce symptoms and improve your quality of life on a daily basis.

Knowledge is power and understanding fosters wisdom. I recommend you read the book, "Virus of the Mind," by Richard Brodie. Not only will it help you understand how your beliefs are created but how to protect yourself from outside forces that can corrupt your mind into believing one thing over another (even when the one thing is not correct or helpful to you).

Chapter 2 will give you a better understanding of where you stand and how to relate to the powerful, potentially life-changing information and action steps provided later in the book.

Chapter Review

- Knowledge truly is power; separating truth from myth is essential to begin your journey to a life free from arthritis pain
- Most people suffer from Osteoarthritis, which is not a disease, but merely a set of symptoms you can manage, overcome and reverse
- You do not have to accept arthritis pain as you age
- You can look healthy and be active, yet still have arthritis
- You can exercise with arthritis, and it will help reduce your symptoms
- You can improve your symptoms through a change in climate or temperature
- Your diagnosis does not sentence you to a wheelchair or nursing home
- You do not have to live in pain; there is hope
- Your arthritis and its symptoms can be reversed; I'll show you how

CHAPTER 2

Arthritis Types and Risk Factors

Arthritis is believed to be the oldest discovered human ailment. Scientists have found this disease in the joints of some dinosaurs and even mummies. The term *arthritis* means "joint inflammation," and the most common types are known as Osteoarthritis (OA) and Rheumatoid arthritis (RA).

Arthritis is a complex family of musculoskeletal disorders consisting of more than 100 different diseases or conditions that destroy joints, bones, muscles, cartilage and other connective tissues, hampering or halting physical movement and causing pain.

Did you know that over 50 million Americans alone have been diagnosed with some form of arthritis? And it's getting worse. Scientists project that by the year 2030, more than 67 million Americans over the age of 18 will be diagnosed with some form of arthritis. These statistics mean that roughly one in five Americans currently deal with the condition.

While arthritis is not a single disease, its symptoms are often universal and are largely experienced as stiffness, soreness, inflammation and pain. Over time, the cartilage between the joints can begin to wear down, exposing the joint to friction. When two bones rub together, inflammation and pain can take place. Redness and swelling of the joints and loss of joint function soon follow.

While the most common form, osteoarthritis, is a result of external factors like physical injury or wear and tear of joints through overuse, this is not the case with rheumatoid arthritis. In fact, despite advances in science, the exact causes of RA are unknown … but certain risk factors have been identified:

- **Genetics** - likely to contribute to risk but no one knows how much.
- **Age** - the older you are the more at risk you become.
- **Weight** – excess weight places a load on the joints that wear them down.
- **Injury** - major injuries are likely to contribute to risk.
- **Occupational Hazards** - repetitive, high-demand jobs increase risk.
- **Sports** - high-level, high-demand sports can contribute to arthritis
- **Illness or infection** - an infection in the joint or gout can lead to arthritis.
- **Stress, Emotions and Beliefs** – how we think, feel and view the world and ourselves can put us at risk for developing arthritis

Let's take a closer look at the two major forms of arthritis and then the solutions you can turn to for relief. Rest assured, no matter what type of arthritis afflicts you, you can find relief with my Arthritis Relief Action Plan.

Osteoarthritis

Osteoarthritis is the degeneration of the cartilage that cushions the area where two bones meet to form a joint. When the cushion wears out or cracks, the bones rub together, causing intense pain. In severe cases, the joints can develop calcifications. This means that calcium builds up on the bones and soft tissues, making them stiff and painful to move. The pain of osteoarthritis gradually worsens with use over the course of the day.

This type of arthritis occurs slowly over time and is the type that many runners, martial artists and construction workers begin to feel by middle age.

Sadly, the most common solution is to relieve the arthritis pain with drugs rather than fixing the problem that is causing the arthritis condition. Research from around the world has proven that there are ways to reverse calcification and to restore damaged cartilage. For those with moderate to severe OA, doing this is the only way to get rid of osteoarthritis pain, once and for all. These solutions are offered in later chapters of this book.

Prevention is always the best medicine. However, reversing damage already done is also essential. Later we will look at the best prevention methods, reversal approaches and lifestyle changes as well as symptomatic relief strategies that are natural and powerful.

Rheumatoid Arthritis

Rheumatoid arthritis, on the other hand, is a chronic disease of the autoimmune system that causes inflammation of the synovial membrane (joint lining). This causes destruction and deformity of bone, cartilage, ligaments and muscle tissue.

RA is a "systemic" disease. Simply put, it affects the whole body. Besides the tissues around the joints, other areas RA affects include the glands of the eyes and mouth, the lining of the lungs and the pericardium (the protective area around the heart). It can reduce both red and white blood cell counts, lowering a person's immune response to viruses and infections. Rheumatoid nodules (hard lumps) can appear around the elbows and fingers, frequently becoming infected. And the most serious complication is blood vessel inflammation, or vasculitis – impairment of the blood supply to the tissues, which leads to tissue death.

Rheumatoid arthritis (RA) is non-discriminating as to whom it affects. Commonly known as "the crippling arthritis," RA's particular symptoms include fatigue, lack of appetite, low-grade fevers, body aches and stiffness. Typically, RA negatively affects several joints at once and in a symmetrical pattern, meaning if the right elbow is inflamed, the left will usually mirror it. Though it can and does attack any joint in the body, RA usually targets the small joints of the hands and feet.

When inflamed, the tissue lining between the joints becomes red, painful and swollen. The frequency and duration of these "flare-ups" vary widely. After repeated episodes, chronic inflammation begins to cause damage to the surrounding tissue, cartilage and bone. Eventually this damage can lead to loss of cartilage and weakening of bones, resulting in painful and permanent destruction and deformities.

The scary and ominous aspect of this disease is the difficulty in diagnosing it – several blood tests (i.e., RF, anti-CCP and ESR) and consideration of signs and symptoms are needed. There isn't one test that doctors can use to determine if someone has RA. Nor do all people with RA display the same set of symptoms. There are cases (approximately 10 percent) where the patient has an immediate initial flare-up. Usually, though, the progress of RA is slow and insidious. Therefore, when the person is finally diagnosed, he or she can already have suffered irreparable damage. Luckily, only one percent of the population suffers RA, and there are solutions to reduce symptoms while stabilizing the immune system to help slow its progression, which will be discussed later in this book.

The traditional course of treatment has been a mixture of rest, exercise and a two-pronged drug therapy attack. While no one would dispute the benefits of relaxation and exercise, the drugs used to treat RA have serious side effects – possibly even death. The sad fact is, they do not even cure the disease. At best, the drugs can mask an RA victim's pain or slow the disease's progress. Even at that, they are not 100 percent effective.

Worldwide research toward finding the cause and cure for RA is very active. At last, the hard work appears to be paying off. Scientists at Case Western Reserve University

(CWRU) carried out two impressive studies. The first shows that a cup of tea – specifically green tea – not only reduces the severity of RA but, in some cases, prevents it all together. The second study offers even more hope as to the healing power of green tea for RA sufferers. Green tea, supplementation and relaxation techniques are powerful solutions for this disease.

Juvenile Arthritis

Sadly, the autoimmune trigger of RA also affects children. In fact, one in 250 American children suffer this disease, known as Juvenile Arthritis (JA). Actually, JA is a term used to group the various autoimmune disorders affecting children 16 and under. While JA affects the joints, it also can affect the eyes, skin and gastrointestinal (GI) tract as well.

JA, while similar to RA, is more easily diagnosed. As a parent or guardian, if a child under your custody or watch complains of or presents swelling in one or more joints for a period of at least six weeks, this may indicate that they have JA. Please take them to see their primary care physician for lab work to know for sure. Again, this autoimmune disease is not precise in how, or whom, it affects, but inherited genes and external factors can trigger it in a child.

The natural solutions and plan for JA are the same as for RA. The difference is that usually a parent or adult will have to manage the lifestyle changes in the home and keep the child on course with the plan.

Please Know There Is Hope!

For me, the worst part about arthritis is that many who have it believe there is no hope for them. They think that because they have arthritis today, they will have it tomorrow. They think that because they experience excruciating pain today, they will experience it tomorrow and keep experiencing it for the rest of their life. It is as if the trajectory of arthritis, to them, is inevitable, and therefore there is no hope. This does not have to be the case. Nothing about arthritis is "inevitable" if you understand the condition and take steps to control it.

Even though this is the case, many don't know it or believe it because of what they have been told. As a result, the Arthritis Foundation reports that a full one-half (50 percent) of Americans suffering with arthritis do not believe anything can be done to help ease their pain. Why? Because the drug-based therapies they have been following are not useful in providing a change to the condition – only symptomatic relief. Yes, immediate relief of pain or stiffness or inflammation is a good thing and drugs are the fastest means for that relief. However, there are two problems with relying on synthetic drug therapies over the long term.

> **Problem 1:** The drugs and cortisone injections are toxic to the system, causing in some cases damage to the liver and stomach lining, weakening of the joint cartilage and the immune system, and GI tract issues.
>
> **Problem 2:** Drugs do not change the course of the condition and thus, as the arthritis worsens

over time, drugs that are more potent are needed, causing more toxicity and potentially damaging side effects.

So, the reliance on synthetic drug therapies cause damage to other parts of the body, and require constant increases in dose, further tearing apart your system. All with little, lasting relief.

The good news is that a multi-pronged approach to arthritis can do wonders, and even feel like a miracle to those suffering its nasty symptoms. Because there is no cure, it is extremely important to become proactive in managing, treating and slowing down the condition. I will say again that by reading this book in the order it is presented, you will gain knowledge and insight into arthritis. This will provide you with understanding and hope. From this, you will be more motivated to approach the various natural solutions and make the necessary lifestyle changes in your life, to improve the quality of your life. *There is hope, and hope is where change begins.*

Chapter Review

- Arthritis affects over 50 million Americans – one in five – and most assume there's no hope
- Osteoarthritis (OA) and Rheumatoid arthritis (RA) are the most common, yet markedly different conditions
- RA is a chronic autoimmune disease causing the joint lining to become inflamed, yet affects **less than one percent** of those with arthritis
- OA is not a disease; it is simply the set of symptoms felt as cartilage in the joints wear down over time, all of which can be prevented and even reversed
- Worsening pain is not inevitable – you can understand the condition and control it with the proper action plan
- You can take steps to prevent or reverse the damage now
- Drug-based therapies set you on a path to worsening health without addressing the real cause of your arthritis
- You can reverse your arthritis with the Arthritis Relief Action Plan – starting now

CHAPTER 3

How Mainstream Medicine Can Make Arthritis Worse

Today more than 150 million Americans suffer chronic pain. This amounts to a whopping 100 percent increase in just a dozen years. How is it possible, with our modern scientific mainstream medicine, that people are suffering more, not less? Clearly, despite their arsenal of elaborate and costly high-tech medical procedures, doctors cannot stop this growing national health emergency.

Part of the reason is because mainstream medicine teaches (trains) people to depend on others for their care after they fall ill. Little is done to help people NOT get sick. Don't believe me? Here are some disturbing statistics:

Arthritis – One in six Americans suffers from arthritis. Twenty-six million of those are women.

Back Pain – It's the leading cause of disability in Americans under age 45. Over 26 million Americans between the ages of 20 and 64 experience frequent back pain, and two-thirds of American adults will have back pain during their lifetime.

Headache – Over 25 million Americans suffer from migraines. Nine out of 10 Americans have non-migraine headaches each year.

As if that were not enough, chronic pain has significant and long-lasting psychological effects. Pain can decrease a person's strength, coordination, independence, cause severe stress and can lead to depression. As a chronic pain sufferer, you will miss an average of four workdays per year and shell out some of the $4 billion spent each year on over-the-counter pain relievers.

Chronic pain has many causes, but frequently the culprits are conditions that cause long-lasting and severe bone, joint and nerve damage. Other factors include falls and accidents, toxins and dehydration, lack of sleep and poor nutrition. In short, these factors cause inflammation and muscle contraction in harmful amounts.

When it comes to pain relief, most people turn first to their medicine cabinet and generally have more than one pain reliever on hand from which to choose. And while pain-relieving drugs (analgesics) are a mainstay of chronic-pain management, the *New England Journal of Medicine* cautions against their side effects: "Long-term use of prescription and over-the-counter nonsteroidal anti-inflammatory drugs (NSAIDs), such as Ibuprofen, can adversely affect a person's digestive tract, liver and kidneys."

A recent study from the University of Pennsylvania Medical Center found that some of the new NSAIDs just recently approved by the FDA might increase the risk of heart attacks, strokes and other harmful cardiovascular problems. Additionally, almost all NSAIDs can cause serious gastrointestinal side effects – including ulceration, bleeding and perforation – at any time and without warning. Not to mention being put at a greater risk of cardiovascular (heart) problems and possible gastrointestinal (stomach and intestine) issues. When it comes to chemical drugs, there are just so many options … and none of them healthy. Let us look at why.

Acetaminophen

While acetaminophen (Tylenol) offers temporary pain relief and fever reduction, it does not reduce swelling (inflammation). It can be harmful to the liver and kidney if you take more than the recommended dose.

Non-Steroidal Anti-inflammatory Drugs (NSAIDs)

Yes, NSAIDs work fast to relieve acute pain, but they may cause gastrointestinal bleeding. They may also be harmful if you have high blood pressure or kidney disease. And they should NEVER be given to children. Aspirin has been associated with onset of a children's disease called Reye's syndrome.

COX-2 Inhibitors

Yes, these work as well as NSAIDs while being less harsh on the stomach, but numerous reports of heart attacks and stroke have prompted the FDA to re-evaluate the risks and benefits of the COX-2s. COX-2 drugs such as Vioxx and Celebrex were actually taken off the market because of these risks.

Disease Modifying Anti-Rheumatic Drugs (DMARDs)

Second-line drugs are called "Disease Modifying Anti-Rheumatic Drugs" (DMARD). These drugs actually address some of the causes of arthritic pain, such as inflammation and swelling. The belief is that their use may help prevent any further damage to the joints. But the price RA victims pay for this "cure" can be very high. Among the least harmful side effects of the more commonly prescribed drug Methodtrexate are headaches, upset stomach, loss of appetite and mouth sores. More dangerous is the drug's potential to reduce the patient's white and red blood cell counts and even to cause kidney damage. Cytoxan, another commonly used DMARD, can increase the risk of developing leukemia and bladder cancer, and can cause temporary or permanent sterility in both men and women.

Narcotics

This class of prescription drugs is powerful, but abuse and addiction are serious side effects. An estimated 20 percent of people in the United States have used prescription drugs for non-medical reasons. The problem is serious and it is growing. The availability of drugs is probably one reason; another is that doctors are prescribing more drugs for more health problems than ever before. And online pharmacies make it easy to get prescription drugs without a prescription, even for youngsters.

The Golden Rule of Pain

When experiencing pain and deciding whether or not to reach for OTC or Rx drugs, please keep in mind that pain and inflammation are not the biggest problem. The biggest problem is simply that **Drugs Don't Heal.** Why? Because arthritis is not caused by a deficiency of drugs. If you are suffering the chronic symptoms of arthritis, then please repeat this mantra:

Drugs don't fix the problem.
Drugs only mask the symptoms.
Pain and inflammation are symptoms,
not diseases.

Many who follow only a scientific medical approach to arthritis end up using supportive devices to remain mobile. They are given drugs, cortisone shots, undergo surgeries and end up still with a cane, then a walker, then must use a wheelchair until their arthritis is so far gone that they need 24-hour assisted care. I don't want this for you. And you don't want this for yourself. Again let me say that the medications and shots and surgeries may help in the short run, but almost always fall short over time to reverse the condition. Please keep an open mind.

When it comes to embracing a natural and all-encompassing arthritis solution, chemical pain relief medications should only be used temporarily, and as needed for breakthrough symptoms while ramping up a natural approach to arthritis, such as the one outlined in this book. The more natural and preventive approach is to understand the pain problem, and take proactive approaches to relieving pain and preventing new pain.

And there are so many options to choose for arthritis relief.

From the work being conducted at Case Western Reserve University (CWRU) and other laboratories, scientists are learning that they don't have to use a sledgehammer to knock out RA. Something as gentle and soothing as a cup of green tea can do the job nicely. I know I mentioned this in the previous chapter. However, I did so to reinforce how something as simple and as natural as a cup of tea has been proven – in a science lab – to be a powerful solution in overcoming a disease mainstream medicine has given up on curing. Let this give you hope, and the effects of prescription drugs scare you just enough, to decide that engaging in the natural approach to overcoming arthritis outlined in this book is worth the lifestyle changes you will need to make to improve your condition and the quality of your life and the ones closest to you.

Chapter Review

- Mainstream medicine offers short-term relief, yet can actually make your arthritis worse
- Many medical doctors throw elaborate and costly procedures at this growing national health emergency – all with little to show for it
- Don't fall victim to the medical myth that you must depend on others for your care
- Golden Rule of Pain: Drugs don't heal; they mask symptoms. You deserve better
- Prescription and over-the-counter drugs are far from safe; they wreak havoc on vital organs without healing the cause of your pain
- Chemical pain medications can help temporarily as you step on the road to natural relief from the Arthritis Relief Action Plan

CHAPTER 4

The 10 Biggest Arthritis Mistakes People Make

No one is perfect, not even doctors. You are human. You are in pain, losing little bits of control and joy from your life each day. It is to be expected that you will make mistakes when it comes to identifying and dealing with your arthritis condition; or in helping a loved one manage theirs. Mistakes are OK when dealing with health and trying to recreate a better quality of life. It's when you don't realize you are making mistakes that real problems occur or that success is lost.

I heard that the definition of insanity is doing the same things repeatedly while expecting different results. When it comes to arthritis, some things work well while others fall short. So doing the same things, making the same mistakes, repeatedly, will definitely not get you to the place you need to be. I would like to take some time here to go over what I see as being the 10 most common, the biggest, mistakes people make when dealing with arthritis. Please read them and see if you may be trapped by them, too. Then let them go and move on to more positive things, a better strategy and start looking toward positive change.

MISTAKE #1

Waiting Too Long to Address Arthritis

Because there is no cure for arthritis, it is especially important that you take steps to prevent it. Once you have been diagnosed, you must become highly proactive in managing, treating and slowing its progression. Reduction of symptoms and changes in lifestyle are essential from the start. It often takes quite a bit of discipline to realize that changing your life (how you work, exercise, eat, etc.) is needed when it comes to overcoming the debilitating nature of this condition. Waiting too long to do something about arthritis is a mistake.

It is one of the biggest mistakes you can make because it allows the condition to take hold and entrench itself in the body, to progress and to wreak havoc. Waiting allows arthritis to steal days and joy from your life. There is no time like the present, so make the decision to begin the rest of your life today by taking control of your arthritis condition.

MISTAKE #2

Undergoing Arthroscopic Surgery

Research that is now widely known and referenced indicates without doubt that arthroscopic surgery to "repair" arthritic joints and the space between them does not work. When it comes to fixing your arthritis condition, it is a mistake to go ahead with physician-recommended arthroscopic surgery. Given the number of years this practice has been in place, I can understand how it is hard to think it a mistake.

While I am not a surgeon, I implore you to listen to the words of Geoffrey Westrich, MD, an orthopedic surgeon at the Hospital for Special Surgery in Manhattan, New York. According to his vast experience, "a doctor who says arthroscopic surgery to repair a torn cartilage or clean out a joint will relieve arthritis pain is doing a huge disservice to a patient. This type of minimally invasive surgery does nothing to relieve arthritis pain … Some patients are actually worse off because their joint becomes inflamed after surgery." So if your primary care physician or orthopedic specialist suggests you do so, please remember it is a mistake and say, "No, thank you."

MISTAKE #3

Avoiding Exercise, Being Sedentary

I know you are in pain and it hurts and is difficult to do what you used to do. I know how much effort it takes to get up and start moving and then to keep moving. Nevertheless, it is a mistake to allow the symptoms of arthritis to keep you from enjoying a vibrant life. In fact, immobility and a sedentary lifestyle are contraindicated when it comes to arthritis. This seems counterintuitive, as you have been told to "rest" your arthritis and to "take it easy." However, the truth is the medical community is now changing its view on this as alternative medicine has been driving home the point that being active, moving around, taking walks and so on reduces the severity of arthritis. How? By lubricating the joints, maintaining their range of motion, improving blood flow, and stabilizing the muscles around arthritis joints.

All of this reduces inflammation and pain as long as the exercise is within a range that you can perform without injury or further damage to your joints. This can only be determined by you, and getting up and exercising a little bit each day, more and more over time, is the way to find out.

MISTAKE #4

Assuming You Won't Get Arthritis If You are "Physically Fit" And "Eat Right"

It takes a lot of effort to get into shape and remain there for prolonged periods. It is important to be healthy and fit. The physically fit and active among us are great at creating a worldview and building a lifestyle around being healthy, fit and vibrant. More people need to do this. A word of caution, however: I would like the fit to know that they are not safe from arthritis. In fact, believing they are immune to such a disorder can be potentially life-disrupting at the inconvenient time it may come on.

You see, RA can come on at any time and for various unknown reasons as it is a result of the immune system being triggered in such a way that it attacks itself. This has nothing to do with how "physically fit" someone may be. While keeping the immune system strong is the best way to prevent such a health event, it is not foolproof. In the case of OA, it is the people who train the hardest, who run and jump the most over prolonged periods, who wear down their joints and damage the cartilage between them. A look at any physical therapy center will show this. There you can see fit athletes (the most highly paid and active professionals among them) in pain, with ice packs and braces, working through their traumas.

The message here is that anyone can suffer arthritis, not just the sedentary and sick. The strong and fit also get arthritis and need to protect against it and manage it in natural ways when it is discovered. It is a mistake to think otherwise.

MISTAKE #5

Not Realizing (or Believing) Diet and Nutrition Play Majors Role in Arthritis

It took a long time for naturalists to gain some respect in America. We have been saying for decades, especially since the 1960s, that diet is essential to health and wellbeing. Yet, the medical profession wanted nothing to do with this idea, saying it did not matter what you put into your mouth. Now after a few decades of tests and discovering things like cholesterol, and finding that the fat stored in your body is the home of toxins, they are changing their stance. You should too, because it is a mistake to believe that diet and nutrition do not play a role in arthritis.

One of the key components of osteoarthritis prevention and reversal is embracing an organic, nutrient-dense diet and taking nutritional supplements to reduce symptoms and shore up wellness. Bone health, joint health, tendon and ligament and muscle health are vital to preventing and reducing the effects of arthritis. Since our bodies are created from the stuff we eat, our cells, blood, and tissues are formed and reformed every seven years based on the quality of our nutritional intake. And when it comes to reducing symptoms, taking natural supplements to reduce inflammation and ease pain and improve joint motility is always easier on the body than taking chemical, artificial drugs. Don't fall victim to the diet and nutrition mistake, instead embrace the advice given in this book, and be proactive about putting good things into your body.

MISTAKE #6

Thinking Doctors and Medical Specialists Have All the Answers

Americans are taught to believe in a healthcare system based in two categories: generalist and specialists. They are taught to see their primary care physician (i.e., "family doctor") with a complaint. If something needs specific attention, patients are sent to the specialist in that field. When it comes to arthritis, the specialist is usually an orthopedist or immunologist.

In either case, it is a mistake to think these people have all the answers; they do not. Yes, they are highly educated in their specific field of treatment, but they are often ignorant of the natural and holistic options and therapies available. Oftentimes, they dismiss such options as hocus pocus. This is a shame because there are dozens and dozens of holistic treatment modalities that are proven effective when attempting to overcome the progression, pain, inflammation and emotional upset of arthritis.

It is important to note, however, that a medical specialist *may* have the right option for you. So keep an open mind in all cases and do look for multiple opinions and resources when considering the path you will take on your road to a better life. And please, don't think the specialists (in any field) have all the answers to your arthritis problems.

MISTAKE #7

Not Giving Natural Therapies Their Due Time

Why don't people use natural therapies as often as toxic and invasive ones? Because they seem to work too slowly or not to work at all. I know how it feels to be in constant pain, to have severely restricted movement, to be inflamed all the time. All you want to do at times like this is to find relief, immediate relief. Oftentimes the fastest route to that relief is drugs, shots and surgeries. But also believe me when I say from experience that these short-term solutions can have some hefty long-term consequences.

Natural therapies like herbal remedies, supplements, dietary changes, energy medicine and manual therapies that gently work the energy lines (meridians), the soft tissue and the skeletal system do work. They work very well, but only when given the time to do their job. Yes, they offer relief but they do so over time. They are gentle and take time to correct the imbalances within the body that cause the arthritis. Drugs only cover the symptoms of the imbalances while doing nothing to correct them. Even though they work quickly, drugs and surgeries have side effects.

Please do not give up on natural therapies and solutions; it is a mistake you may later regret. Give them time to do what they do in a natural way. It is a mistake just to "try" them for a short period, or even a single time, and say they don't work because they didn't meet your expectation of immediate relief. Instead, change your expectation to echo that of the provider or product and then settle in and give it time to make the lasting changes it is meant to create.

MISTAKE #8

Continuing on a Treatment Plan That's Not Working

Keeping mistake number seven in mind, it is just as serious a mistake to keep doing the things that are proving unsuccessful for you. If you give a natural remedy the time necessary to work as it should, and it falls short for you or does not seem to help you, then it is a mistake to keep doing it. On the same note, continuing along a plan of medication to mask symptoms of arthritis that is not successful in altering the condition in a positive way is a mistake; discontinue it.

This book alone should provide you the knowledge that there are nearly a hundred options for overcoming arthritis. Read the entire book and consider which may be best for you, and in which combinations, then give it the best effort you can. If after three months of diligently following a protocol, (IF you do it properly), and you are not feeling better or headed in that direction, change course a bit and implement the other options in the book. It is a mistake to continue doing what is not working for you because it is stealing time from your life. Move on to the next one and find the mix of products and therapies and practices that, when combined, do what you need them to. Everyone is different. After all, healing is an art, not a science.

MISTAKE #9

Believing There Are No More Options Left

Having been a chronic pain sufferer myself, I know that you have been through the mill when it comes to finding some relief from the chronic and daily suffering that goes along with arthritis. You will recall from the end of Chapter 2 that we discussed the need for hope and that there is plenty of hope when it comes to most cases of arthritis. This notion is so important to a successful outcome of the natural arthritis program outlined in this book that I wanted to be clear. Believing there are no options left – that you have exhausted all options within the medical profession for arthritis relief – is a mistake.

There are so many causes and triggers for arthritis and the symptoms associated with it. And the good news is that within the treasure chest of alternative medicine and holistic therapies are hundreds of options that can work for you. Please read this book carefully and find the ones that seem to speak to you and your arthritic condition. We are all different and require a unique approach, a different blend of the means and methods. Despite what the medical establishment tells you, there is no one-size-fits-all approach to arthritis. That is why what you have been doing there has not worked. If it had, you would not be reading this book. But you are, and hope is found within the options presented herein.

MISTAKE #10

Failing To Take Personal Control of Your Situation

The most powerful thing you can ever come to know is the fact that no one cares about your arthritis condition as much as you do. They simply do not have as big a stake in it. You are the one suffering, not them, so to rely on others to take care of your condition is a big mistake. You must take personal control of your arthritis. It is only you who can change your lifestyle, removing the things that negatively affect your health and wellness. It is only you who can eat right and take supplements and administer pain relieving creams and gels. It is only you who can stretch, walk, exercise and meditate. So please find a way to become self-empowered and to take control. I know it is hard. I struggle with it, too. But if you don't do it, who will? And to help you find that passion for change and to develop the self-empowered spirit I have included material on motivation toward the end of the book. You can do it. I know you can!

Chapter Review

- We all make mistakes when it comes to identifying and dealing with arthritis
- Understanding, learning from, and avoiding these mistakes start your journey to a life free from arthritis pain
- Save yourself time and pain by avoiding the 10 most common mistakes
- Three mistakes come from **inaction**:
    - Waiting too long
    - Avoiding exercise
    - Expecting others to take control
- Five mistakes come from **misinformation**:
    - Ignoring diet's ability to prevent or reverse symptoms
    - Assuming physical fitness alone prevents symptoms
    - Relying only on doctors for answers or cures
    - Expecting arthroscopic surgery to work
    - Continuing a failing plan because it should work
- The last two mistakes come from **giving up**:
    - Tossing aside natural therapies too quickly
    - Believing there are no solutions

CHAPTER 5

How Inflammation Keeps You from Healing

Most people experience more than one health concern at a time. Very rarely do people suddenly encounter an isolated issue like low back pain or diseases like Alzheimer's, cancer and arthritis. Generally, they have an underlying condition in the body that precedes and, indeed, causes or contributes to the "sudden" health concern that arises.

In many cases, it is the same condition within the body that allows pain, illness and disease to take hold, making us feel unwell. That underlying condition is *chronic low-grade inflammation*. Inflammation plays two nasty roles in arthritis.

Pain is certainly a major symptom of arthritis. However, pain is generally felt as a reaction to swelling or inflammation in the body. This efferent signal is the body's way of telling you something is wrong and in need of change. Inflammation, then, is both a sign and a symptom of pain.

The term "inflammation" generally evokes thoughts of painful joints and muscles, swelling and loss of mobility. These are the obvious markers of inflammation, but research also shows that chronic inflammation, if left untreated, can actually lead to serious diseases, including diabetes, heart disease, some cancers and Alzheimer's.

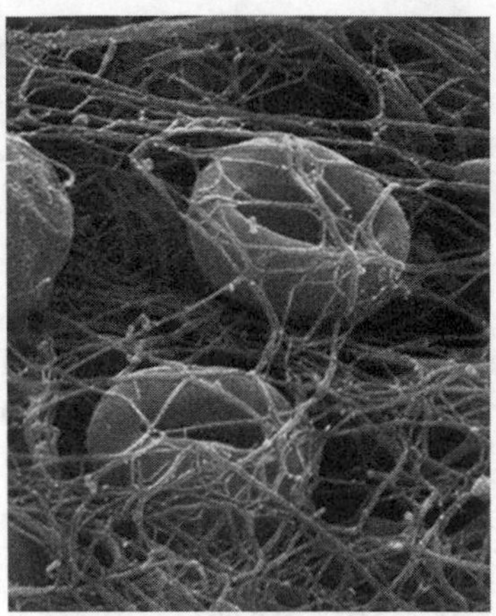

The amount of inflammation in your body varies and is dependent on a number of factors – including your activity level, the amount of sleep you get, the degree of stress in your life, and yes … even the food you eat. What you have to realize is that these factors are cumulative; they build up over time. And the more that any or all of these factors become out of control, the risk for disease increases.

If you have pain due to inflammation, which you do if you have arthritis, you may choose to take the traditional medical path, which includes non-steroidal anti-inflammatory drugs (NSAIDs), steroids, cortisone injections and even go so far as to have joint-replacement surgery. But as you will learn in the following chapters in this book, none of these "big guns" may be necessary. You should especially avoid long-term use of prescription and over-the-counter anti-inflammatory painkillers.

These have been proven to cause liver dysfunction, kidney failure, stomach bleeding and ulcer … all causes of additional inflammation.

Please keep in mind that inflammation is not a disease. However, because so many health problems have been associated with it, it's tempting to think of inflammation as a disease. And of course inflammation is not always a bad thing. It's a vital part of a healthy immune response. Your body depends on inflammatory responses to defend you from bacterial and viral invaders and even cancer cells. Inflammation also helps the body heal from injuries.

When You Need To Worry

Inflammation is a natural response your body has to stress. However, inflammation that is chronic and low-grade or not externally apparent is cause for concern. That kind of inflammation may show as a skin redness or rash, but it may also present as chronic pain or fever.

Inflammation that remains in the body can wreak havoc, causing serious health concerns and disease. It is caused and remains active because of genetics, diet, lifestyle choices and one's environment. Chronic inflammation breaks your body's internal balance point, disrupts its ability to regulate the immune system and affects the functions of the central nervous system. Under the influence of chronic low-grade inflammation, you run a greater risk for pain, stiffness and other symptoms associated with arthritis. With regard to RA, keeping inflammation at bay is vital.

Signs and Symptoms of Inflammation

You should always be mindful of the state of your health and wellness. If you find you experience chronic conditions that could be described as "annoyances" and don't require an immediate trip to your doctor, then keep an eye on them. If these irritating signs and symptoms remain for more than a month (some linger for years, even decades, if not treated), you may be experiencing chronic low-grade inflammation. Signs, symptoms, conditions and diseases associated with inflammation include: acid reflux, acne, arthritis, asthma, autoimmune diseases, bronchitis, cancer, candidiasis, diabetes, fatigue, fever, gout, headache, heart disease, high blood pressure (HBP), infections, join pain, neuropathy, osteoporosis, psoriasis, sciatica, stiffness, swelling and urinary tract infections (UTI).

I recommend working with your doctor or health care provider to assess your level of systemic inflammation. One of the key ways of determining this is through a blood test that measures the level of C-reactive protein (CRP) in your blood. CRP shows up in higher amounts when there is inflammation in the body. Usually, the inflammation tested for follows surgical procedures or an infection you may have had. However, because of diet, stress and lifestyles many people have systemic low-grade inflammation all the time. Knowing this will help you understand your condition and embrace the solutions in this book.

Please believe me when I tell you that stress is one of the major, yet least talked about, causes of inflammation. Not only that, the negative effects of stress take their toll on all aspects of your life and well-being, including reducing your life span. There are many stressors that affect you and that you need to be aware of.

Emotional Stressors can have many causes. These include a poor relationship with your significant other and tense relationships at the office. Internal struggles with self-worth and achievement of personal goals are other examples of how psychological conflicts can stress the body, leading to inflammation, muscle tightness, constricted blood flow and overstimulation by the central nervous system.

Physical Stressors are perhaps the most obvious causes of inflammation. Working out too hard or for too long without proper warm-up can cause muscle strains and joint sprains. Pain, redness and swelling along the muscles or around the joints are the sure signs. In these cases, short-term inflammation is desirable, but prolonged inflammation is unhealthy and must be reduced and eliminated.

Dietary Stressors can wreak havoc on the body through impairing digestion, hindering waste motility, promoting abdominal distension and causing acid reflux. Diets that are high in fat and cholesterol, refined flour and sugar, diuretic beverages containing caffeine and alcohol, and allergens like nuts can cause chronic inflammation that may go unnoticed until a major problem occurs.

Subtle Stressors

Environmental stressors are perhaps the hardest to detect or attribute to personal health. Yet living or work environments that are damp or mildewed inflame the lungs and sinuses. Fluorescent lamps, power lines and electronic devices (especially wireless) attack the body with damaging electromagnetic frequencies.

Lifestyle choices are the stressors that are most amenable to control and alleviation. These include not eating right, skimping on sleep, indulging in recreational drugs, relying on pharmaceuticals while avoiding natural solutions and harboring negative feelings. This list also includes watching too much television or engaging in too much physical activity when the body is not prepared for it.

Since this is such an important aspect of the program, more detailed information on stress, emotions and the mind/body connection are provided in Chapters 7, 16 and 17.

Natural Methods to Reduce Inflammation

It is very important to reduce and eliminate chronic low-grade inflammation to allow the body to restore its internal balance. When the body is left to its restorative ways and not interrupted or prevented by inflammation, there is a good chance of attaining a healthy state of wellness. When the body is out of balance, the risk for developing inflammatory-related signs, symptoms, conditions and diseases increases. The good news is that there are plenty of simple, natural ways to reduce inflammation and take control of your health.

These include reducing your stress, improving your diet, exercising in balance, balancing lifestyle and taking supplementation. Each of these is covered in much more detail in the next sections of the book.

The problem is one of balance (more on this in Chapter 8). Because of poor diet and lifestyle, our bodies tend to over-produce inflammatory chemicals. At the same time, we don't get enough of the nutrients that naturally reduce inflammation. If you are carrying around a few extra pounds, your risk of inflammation-related illness is magnified. Fat cells produce inflammatory chemicals at a rate far greater than other cells. When you gain weight (or fail to lose it), you are putting your body under an additional inflammatory burden that increases your risk of disease and accelerates the aging process. The threat is double-edged, because excessive inflammation also makes it difficult for you to lose weight.

Healthy lifestyle habits such as exercising regularly, not smoking, maintaining a healthy weight and minimizing stress all help to reduce inflammation. One of the biggest factors in chronic low-level inflammation may be the food you eat every day and an acidic internal body environment.

Chapter Review

- Chronic low-grade inflammation is often the root of many health concerns, especially arthritis and pain
- While inflammation is your body's natural response to stressors, ignoring the issue can lead to serious diseases and long-term consequences
- Inflammation is dependent upon stress, your activity level, the amount of sleep you get, and the food you eat
- Reduce and eliminate chronic low-grade inflammation through stress reduction, appropriate exercise, balanced diet and lifestyle, and critical dietary supplements

CHAPTER 6

How Food Impacts Arthritis

One of the difficult things that many struggle with in their lives is frustration with food. Overweight people are looking to shed pounds. Skinny people are looking to bulk up. Those looking to detox or just to be healthy are vying for non-genetically modified organisms (GMO), organic foods. New books and programs and studies on diets throw us all for loops. It's so confusing to be in the food store and get lost in all the claims about what is healthy and not healthy for you. So you make your way to a vitamin shop or Whole Foods and try your luck there. But when you grab a bag of this, or a bar of that, and turn it to read the label … you are just as lost. In this chapter, I would like to discuss in simple terms how your food choices can exponentially increase how arthritis impacts you.

Excess Weight Contributes to Arthritis

Those who are overweight and suffering arthritis of the hips or knees or feet must slim down. Period. Overweight and obesity are among the most serious risk factors for arthritis. And being overweight is a condition that many can control. I am not passing judgment about your self-image or the emotional issues that may be leading you to overindulge in food. I am speaking simply of the fact that when arthritic, the joints of the body are stressed, inflamed, swollen and painful. As such, excess weight can both contribute to the cause of osteoarthritis and to the worsening of its symptoms.

This obesity situation affects you in two debilitating ways:

- The extra weight can cause a great load on the joint and wear away the cartilage over time to contribute to, or cause, arthritis.

- People who are overweight tend to have less energy and are less likely to be or remain physically active, which worsens the arthritis condition.

According to the Centers of Disease Control (CDC), 54 percent of arthritis sufferers are, indeed, obese. "People who have a higher body mass index tend to get arthritis earlier in life," they warn. "Additionally, if they require joint replacement surgery, their new joints tend to wear out during their lifetime because they are younger and therefore have more years to live than the traditional joint replacement patient."

What I would like you really to understand is that the excess weight you carry around places a compressive-load on your joints that is three times the actual weight. That means for every 15 pounds you are overweight, your hips and knees are under stress to move a 45-pound load. If you are 30 to 40 or more pounds overweight … you do the math. It is staggering.

Consider for a minute the other end of the weight issue. According to the research of Stephen Messier, PhD of

Wake Forest University, and published in the journal *Arthritis & Rheumatism*, "For people losing 10 pounds, each knee would be subjected to 48,000 pounds less in compressive load per mile walked." That is a huge amount of potential prevention – and relief from arthritis symptoms – with a relatively small loss of excess weight.

Please take weight as a serious factor in your condition. If you are overweight, and more than half of you reading this book are, please take steps to decrease your body mass. I will help you and have outlined the way in Chapter 10.

Food Can Cause Pain and Inflammation

When it comes to pain and inflammation, the food you consume plays a role. You see, food is a critical piece of the puzzle when it comes to controlling for these life and energy draining symptoms. Unfortunately, the typical American diet consists of too much fat, tons of sugar, loads of red meat and a frightening amount of processed foods. Is it a wonder there are so many people suffering arthritis? These foods cause inflammation, block the bowels, drain the immune system and deplete the blood of dense nutrients. When it comes to arthritis, several categories of food should be avoided, including nightshades, milk-based products and high-fructose corn syrup (HFCS).

The nightshade fruits and vegetables are particularly troublesome for those suffering with arthritis. This family of food includes white potatoes, eggplant, sweet and hot peppers, tomatoes, tomatillos, tamarios, pepinos, pimentos, goji berries, ground cherries, Cape gooseberries, garden huckleberries and paprika.

These foods can cause calcification, bone spurs and inflammation. These side effects are deleterious to those suffering arthritis. In cases of people who are sensitive or allergic to nightshades, they can cause nerve damage, muscle tremors and impeded digestion.

Milk-based products are also troublesome for those suffering with arthritis. They are often high in cholesterol and saturated fat, and so can contribute to obesity. And as we learned, being overweight by even 15 pounds can have disastrous effects on arthritic joints. Secondarily, products like milk, yogurt, ice cream, cheese, cottage cheese and various sauces can contribute to an increase in phlegm-rheum. Phlegm-rheum is a classification of thick, sticky fluids in the body that include mucus. These thick and sticky fluids pool around joints and collect toxins, bacteria and become either damp or hot, depending on other factors. This increases inflammation, swelling, bone degeneration, loss of range of motion and pain. One of the things you will learn about in the book is how to dry the body of such sticky fluids to improve circulation, reduce swelling and inflammation and decrease pain.

The sweetener known as high fructose corn syrup (HFCS) has been called the main culprit in the rise in youth obesity in the United States, and as we discussed obesity is one of the key risks for arthritis. High-fructose corn syrup is corn syrup that has undergone enzymatic processing to convert its glucose into fructose. This fructose has then been mixed with regular corn syrup, which is 100 percent glucose, and the result is a sweet liquid known as high-fructose.

This liquid is the sweetener found in just about every cold beverage in your local convenience store, including iced tea, sodas and energy drinks. Not only that, but it is also found in so-called healthy foods like tomato soup and yogurt, and less healthful items such as salad dressings and cookies. The FDA did a 30-year study and found a correlation between HFCS and obesity, stating that it is worse for your health than plain sugar – which also is not good for those with pain and inflammation.

Acidic Food Negatively Affect Arthritis

I know it may sound strange, but your body, your body fluids and your blood can become acidic. What does that mean? You know how acidic fruits like lemons, can "eat" the enamel off your teeth and how acids can corrode a battery casing? Well, your body can become overly acidic, too, when the natural pH or ratio of acid to base (alkaline) is off kilter.

The initials pH refer to the scientific term "potential hydrogen." This is the concentration of hydrogen ions in the body. The pH falls into a range of 0-14, with the sweet spot for human blood being around 7.35. As the numbers increase, the body is becoming more alkaline, but when the numbers decrease it indicates the body is becoming more acidic. Being in a constant or chronic acidic state is not only unhealthy it is damaging to the body.

The human body was not designed to withstand chronic acidic states. When the body is off-kilter long enough, out of its natural state of homeostasis, it starts to break down. Signs and symptoms of an excessively acidic body can be seen and/or felt externally, with the onset of headaches, body pain and skin rashes. In the acidic range, the immune system is compromised, leading to easily contracted sinus infections, allergies, cold and flu, and place you at risk for progressing autoimmune diseases, rheumatoid arthritis (RA). Moreover, an acidic interior environment can lead to muscle contraction that can restrict the free flow of blood and inhibit the exchange of nutrients and waste products from muscle cells. This can cause soreness, cramping, fatigue, degenerative cellular diseases and even cellular death.

pH Balance Guide

Acid	0	Battery Acid
	1	Stomach Acid
	2	Lemon Juice, Vinegar
	3	Orange Juice, Soda
	4	Tomato Juice, Beer
	5	Black Coffee
	6	Saliva, Cow's Milk
Neutral	7	Pure Water
Alkaline	8	Sea Water
	9	Baking Soda
	10	Antacid
	11	Ammonia
	12	Soapy Water
	13	Bleach, Oven Cleaner
	14	Drain Cleaner

Arthritis, or "inflammation of the joints," is related to pH imbalance and accumulation of acid deposits in the joints of the neck, hips, wrists and hands. It is the accumulated acid that damages cartilage. When the cells that produce the lubricating synovial fluids and bursa fluids are acidic, this condition causes a dryness that irritates and swells the joints. When uric acid builds up it tends to deposit in the form of crystals that can feel like broken glass in the feet, hands, knees and back.

Thankfully, you don't have to worry about this when your body is kept within the alkaline range of 7.0 - 7.4. In fact, while in this range it is impossible for disease to sustain itself because the immune system is strong and there is no longer an acidic environment necessary for diseases, like cancer, gout and arthritis. This chart will help you see just how the foods you eat and the beverages you drink contribute to an unhealthy internal environment.

An imbalanced pH or acid/alkaline interior environment is *one of the hidden causes of arthritis* and one of the states that makes it symptoms worse. How does the body become too acidic and thus unhealthy and place you at risk for negative health symptoms, like those associated with arthritis? Well, stress is a big one. Stress, or the effects of being in the "fight or flight" response for too long a period of time, releases stress hormones into the body, flooding the blood stream with protective chemicals. These chemicals, like cortisol, were necessary during the times of our great ancestors who had to run for their lives from wild beasts or head hunting tribes. These days, the stress response happens from different types of stressors, like emotional upset, physically demanding work and overwhelming psychological issues that we deal with at home and work. There are too many of these happening throughout the day. It is no wonder we are under chronic states of stress, are not well and are in constant acidic states. Dealing with stress is huge when it comes to reducing the symptoms of arthritis. In Chapter 16, I will show you how to do it, naturally.

Our modern diet is also a huge contributor to our chronic acidic interior environment. When food reaches your digestive tract, it is broken down and either leaves an alkaline or an acidic residue behind. If one eats foods that are organic, whole and fresh and drinks plenty of pure water the body can easily maintain an alkaline state. However, consuming sugar, refined grains, preservatives, pesticides, dairy products like cow's milk, cheese, yogurt and ice cream, red meat, chocolate, coffee, soda and alcohol turns the body acidic. One of the main culprits of poor diet is inflammation, which is also the main symptom of arthritis and pain.

As I mentioned, pH is a measure of the potential hydrogen or residue a food leaves behind, as either being alkaline or acidic. And this is not directly related to the acidic nature of a food before it is digested. Lemons, for example, are highly acidic. If you squeeze the juice of a lemon on an open wound, it will burn. However, when ingested and digested, lemon is very alkalizing for the body and lemon juice can help reduce acidic levels. A diet that is low in acidic foods and packed full of nutrient-dense alkalizing foods will make you healthier while also reducing the symptoms of arthritis. This diet is explained later in the book.

If you have arthritis, suffer symptoms like pain and stiffness, and have a predisposition to infection it is likely that an imbalanced pH is present in your body. To be sure, you can purchase pH testing strips or rolls in your local drug store. These are thin paper items that gauge your pH level when dipped either into your saliva or urine stream, first thing in the morning before anything is eaten or drunk. What you want is each day to be in either the alkaline range or moving toward it.

Natural methods of reducing the acidic environment in your body in favor of alkalizing it will be shared on the chapters dealing with diet, supplements and mind/body techniques. In the meantime, please control this unhealthy environment by avoiding or severely restricting the foods mentioned in this chapter.

In Chapter 10, I will discuss how to eat for healthy weight reduction, a pro-alkaline and anti-inflammatory environment and for joint health. It is important to view food in terms of how it affects the body. It can make it strong or weak – that is, every structure, bones, tendons, muscles, tissues. Arthritis affects all of these, so a diet that is anti-inflammatory, free of chemical pesticides and nutrient dense while also providing a boost to blood flow and the feel good hormones is what you will want to embrace. I will tell you the how and why and show you how to put it into place. Until then, and in the meantime, please be mindful of the harmful effects certain foods and beverages can have, not only on your arthritic condition, but also on your emotional state and quality of life.

Chapter Review

- Obesity and excess weight is one of the most serious, debilitating factors in arthritis symptoms – increasing stress on joints and diminishing energy and physical activity
- Food can cause pain and inflammation – giving you the power to improve your arthritis symptoms through diet
- Avoid fatty, sugary, and processed foods to stave off pain and inflammation
- Monitor your internal pH to keep your body from harboring an acidic environment – a step that is critical to improving pain from inflammation
- Your diet is an important part of the solution to achieving a life free from arthritis pain

CHAPTER 7

How Stress and Emotions Affect Arthritis

The content of your mind and the state of your emotions play a vital role in both wellness and illness. While emotions are natural and important parts of life, in excess they can be damaging to the body. Where arthritis is concerned, many suffering the disease of RA and the condition of OA suffer stress, mental and emotional fatigue and depression. Often times these emotional states are a result of having the arthritis condition itself. What is even worse is that these states of being can cause pain and inflammation to worsen and lead to feelings of hopelessness.

Please believe me when I tell you that *this does not need to be the case*. Something more can be done and in many cases a lot more can be done to help you. Reading this chapter in itself will help because it can put your arthritis and its symptoms in context of your thoughts and feelings. Once you come to see how mind and emotions, often directed by stress, affect you for better or worse, you will be able to embrace more fully the mind-body techniques explored later in the book. These will be of tremendous help to you in overcoming the severity of your arthritic condition.

When it comes to conditions like arthritis, the mind and emotions hold key positions in how you experience the condition and in the potential outcomes of a program for relief. Understanding this and getting on top of it is a key component of finding relief and deriving a better quality of life. Let us look at why this is the case.

The Mind-Body Connection

Stress erodes your health and undermines your quality of life. It is a psychosomatic response to what is happening around you. That is to say, it is a physical manifestation in the body of what the mind perceives and struggles with.

In decades past, the term psychosomatic was primarily used by psychologists to identify pain or illnesses that were assumed to be "all in the mind" of the patient and, therefore, "not real." This outlook is dated and false. The seed of the physical condition *is* in the thoughts and emotions of the person affected by them. However, these symptoms are not "imaginary," but felt in the body in very real ways. Indeed, they exist in very real forms, like inflammation, swelling, spasms, trigger points, pain and depression.

The answer to the puzzle of how the mind affects the body and the body affects the mind may well be found within the mind itself, and the hold it has over your thoughts, emotions and the quality of your physical body. When the mind (psycho) and the body (soma) come together in adverse ways to manifest pain, inflammation, rashes, muscle spasms … it is called psychosomatic illness. This is just a technical way of saying there is a direct connection and relationship between your mind and your body.

The mind-body (psychosomatic) connection is a real two-way street. Your mind affects your body and your body affects your mind. How?

Well, when you think your condition is bad and that nothing can be done, you release stress hormones that negatively affect your health over time and your feelings of well-being in the moment. These then create negative cycles of stress and anxiety that can lead to depression. These emotions decrease your energy, slow your breathing, decrease your blood flow and make you unmotivated to get up and move. This causes muscle tightness, weight gain, loss of range of motion, inflammation and pain.

You see, it is interrelated. When your body feels in pain or cannot do what you ask of it, this affects your mind and emotions. When your mind and emotions are too negative you begin to feel worse, experience more pain and stop doing things you used to enjoy. This causes more of the symptoms that make your condition feel worse and deteriorate it faster. Stress plays a large role in this.

The Stress Response

It all starts with stress derived from worry about your arthritic condition, the loss of activity and joy in the present and how you will fare in the years to come. Stress and worry are major components of how you perceive your pain and arthritis situation and, also, of how your arthritic symptoms manifest.

Please don't feel bad about this. You are not alone. Stress is one of the leading causes of illness in the United States. Nearly 66 percent of all signs and symptoms presented in doctors' offices in the U.S. are stress induced. And the symptoms most associated with arthritis are known to be aggravated and often severely increased by stress.

What happens when you are under stress – real or perceived – is that your body moves through a *stress response*. Through the physiological mechanism of stress, your muscles tighten, which inhibits circulation and constricts blood vessels, causing stiffness, trigger points, inflammation, limited range of motion and pain. The hypertonic (painfully tight) muscles place a compressive load on the arthritic joints and the trigger points slow the flow of blood and thus the exchange of blood, oxygen and nutrients. Toxins then remain in the muscle tissue, collect in the thick fluids in and around the joints, and cause swelling, inflammation and pain.

The effects of stress include nail biting, anxiety, a racing mind, obsessive thoughts, compulsive behavior, unending worry, muscle tension and spasm, poor appetite, over eating, digestive disorders, constipation, insomnia, poor blood flow, belabored breathing, neck pain, shoulder tension and the possible onset or continuation of bad habits such as dependence on alcohol, drugs, painkillers, food and caffeine.

The Nasty Cycle

While this is all normal, it is not necessary to maintain. In fact, when left unchecked, stress actually triggers a cycle of worry about those symptoms, which then makes your arthritic condition and its symptoms worse. Round and round it goes until stress, anxiety and depression become the dominant mental framework and emotional set point. This can make you feel like your condition is helpless, that nothing can be done to improve it, and that you will live an unhappy life that is severely hampered.

Again, these mental and emotional states have a negative impact on the nervous system and take their toll on the body. Without adequate blood flow, the cells in your body become slightly oxygen deprived. Toxins and waste aren't cleaned out as efficiently as they should be and can build up in certain parts of your body, creating or reactivating trigger points. These knots are often painful to the touch and, in some cases, can cause muscles to spasm or "lockup," which can compress your arthritic joints, causing even greater pain, inflammation, restricted range of motion, stress, frustration and depression.

Without fresh blood supplying oxygen and nutrients, it is nearly impossible to heal. Stress also alters your breathing. Typically, when you are anxious or upset, your breath becomes shallow, reducing oxygen flow to the whole body. Oxygen and nutrients don't circulate at optimum levels, again contributing to the buildup of toxins. Stress also can release hormones, such as adrenaline - which can trigger chronic tension and inflammation in your muscles, ligaments and tendons - and increased levels of cortisol which causes fat to accumulate across your midsection affecting heart health and increases your chances of becoming overweight (which as you will recall places a tremendous burden on the joints). Without adequate blood flow to remove these hormones from the body, they can linger longer than usual and create more damage.

The effect of such prolonged or recurring stress is that it keeps the autonomic nervous system from balancing, which can lead to problems with the gastrointestinal tract, the digestive system, the respiratory system and the neuroendocrine system. When coupled with arthritis, stress can also lead to depression, which can lock in an almost permanent negative mental and emotional state that can be hard to overcome.

Depression affects more than 20 million Americans and represents a serious mental health problem. It is believed to involve a genetic predisposition and the chemical composition of the brain, where symptoms like loss of energy, fatigue, prolonged feelings of deep sadness, loss of interest in things and even thoughts of suicide stay front and center for an extended period.

Many folks treat depression with psychotherapy or prescription antidepressant drugs. Although many experts think a combination of these two are effective, no scientific evidence supports this supposition. In reality, research shows that simple, natural measures like more sleep, exercise, supplementation, diet and efforts at *sustaining a positive attitude work better to combat depression than medication.*

What You Think Becomes Your Reality

A lot has been written lately about the Law of Attraction. The works of Abraham-Hicks, Wayne Dyer, Deepak Chopra and Eckhart Tolle have given people a better understanding of the way in which our minds not only affect but create our perceptions and our lives. If perception is reality, then what you think (the content of your mind) forms your belief system. Your belief system affects how you then see the world and how you in turn respond to it. This includes your perception of arthritis and how it does and will affect you.

The mind is inextricably connected to the body. If you want to be healthy and happy instead of in pain and feeling sick, you have to readjust your attitude toward health. Healthy people are happy people. And shifting your attitude from "nothing helps" to "I can make better choices" is often the key step that offers optimal wellness and emotional fulfillment. Health and happiness represent a frame of mind that influences your choices. Making better lifestyle choices leads to wellness and a better quality of life.

It is therefore necessary and actually vital that you work toward thinking positively about yourself, your life and your arthritis condition. Let your emotions be your guide in self-regulating the stress and its mind-body cycle. When you feel bad, reframe your mind with the techniques taught in Section II. Looking for and finding the positive in all aspects of your life will attract more positive thoughts and feelings. These will decrease the stress and anxiety of arthritis, help stave off depression and keep you as active as you can be. This will help you better follow the program outlined in Section III and swipe away the negative impact on the arthritic conditions you feel.

Chapters 16 and 17 present dozens of natural and proven methods and strategies for combating the emotional distress and stress of arthritis, in addition to treatment methods and self-help modalities and items for overcoming arthritis. Take some time to review Section I, then begin Section II with a fresh mind and invigorated spirit.

Chapter Review

- Don't let your pain be worsened by stress and mental and emotional fatigue
- Understand your mind and body are intricately connected; negative emotions increase your pain and multiply your physical symptoms
- Simply by readjusting your attitude toward health and your arthritis condition in a positive way, you can experience improvement
- Let your emotions be your guide in self-regulating stress and the mind-body cycle
- Read Section II for techniques to reframe your mind toward better health

CHAPTER 8

The 3 Hidden Imbalances That Cause Arthritis

The secret of overcoming arthritis is to understand where it begins. The Arthritis Relief Action Plan is built on correcting the three hidden imbalances that derail your health and actually cause pain, illness and diseases like arthritis. These hidden imbalances are the beginnings or root causes that must be understood before you can create a program for relieving them. You can then make changes in your lifestyle that make it better and create balance to prevent the symptoms of arthritis from running roughshod over your life.

The causes of arthritis are seemingly many, yet they all have something in common: they are based in a combination of one of three types of imbalance. These imbalance categories are known as **Excesses** (too much of something), **Deficiencies** (too little of something) and **Stagnation** (things moving too slowly). For short, I will refer to this concept simply as EDS (excess/deficiency/stagnation). To understand what is meant by these terms, let us first consider *homeostasis* – the body's natural state of balance.

THE BASELINE OF HEALTH

Homeostasis is the body's baseline of health and well-being. It is the state where you feel good, not too stressed, tired or excited. You are in a state where your digestion is working properly, your body is absorbing proper amounts of nutrients and oxygen and is expelling toxins through the skin, lungs and intestines. Your sleep and wake cycle is set, you work and exercise, you have a balanced home-work-social life. Things are good.

But life often gets in the way and we don't feel as good anymore. Poor health, pain and disease are all felt in the body when it is off balance or is no longer functioning at homeostasis. This happens when you experience or engage in excesses (e.g., too much alcohol or exercise), deficiencies (e.g., not enough sleep or too little exercise) or stagnations (e.g., muscle spasms or constipation).

People suffer needlessly every day because they and their healthcare practitioners operate from a disease-based model of health. "Mr. Smith, you have arthritis pain, so we will treat the pain of the arthritis." This approach does not work, obviously, because millions of people still suffer from the pain of arthritis.

I propose that you view your overall health, your arthritis condition and its symptoms in particular, as examples of imbalance.

Explaining the EDS Puzzle

The three terms that comprise EDS revolve around the idea that to slow the progress of your arthritis and to live as symptom-free as possible, you need to maintain a balance within and between your body, your mind and your diet. In other words, you need to make changes to your lifestyle. It is important to avoid too much (i.e., excess) of anything that causes your condition or its symptoms to get worse, or too little (i.e., deficiency) of something to prevent it from getting better. Let's take a look at this concept of "three hidden causes" as associated with the connection between your body/mind/diet (i.e., lifestyle) and arthritis.

Arthritis Excesses

Too much of even a good thing can be bad. That is a popular saying that is certainly true when it comes to arthritis. When we consider how osteoarthritis develops, we will see it is from wear and tear on the joint structures.

This is often the result of too much (or an excess of) exercise; at least the wrong kind. As stated earlier in the book, exercise is needed to help reduce the symptoms of arthritis. Yet, too much of rigorous forms like martial arts, long-distance running and aerobics can lead to breakdown of the cartilage and compression of the joints, leading to an arthritic condition.

A diet that is in excess of fructose and carbohydrates is also detrimental to arthritis because it leads to becoming overweight and possibly to obesity. As we learned earlier, over half of all arthritis sufferers are obese. What's more, even a relatively small number of pounds over a healthy weight can cause a compressive force three times their measure. Thus, a diet that includes too many sweets, carbohydrates, alcohol, dairy products and nightshades are detrimental to the formation of and aggravate the symptoms associated with arthritis.

Emotions, as we learned in the previous chapter, play a big role in your arthritis experience. First, some have a mindset for success that leads them to push, push, push to get things done, to run the extra mile, to eat while working and then forgo rest and relaxation. This Type A personality can actually contribute to getting both forms of arthritis. The excessive pushing behavior wears down the body (and can lead to osteoarthritis) and the immune system (which can lead to rheumatoid arthritis).

The next part is the preponderance (excess) of low-vibration emotions that comes once you have been diagnosed with arthritis. Wallowing in sorrow for too long, chronically feeling that nothing can be done and complaining to everyone are all ways in which an excess of negative emotion can derail progress. Arthritis can feel worse than it is and can progress more rapidly when you embrace a life excessively ripe with negative thoughts, feelings and emotions.

Arthritis Deficiencies

When it comes to arthritis, deficiencies also play a role in both cause and relief. If you have a diet that lacks the appropriate amount of whole, fresh fruits and vegetables, you are depriving your body of the nutrients necessary for growth and strength. Blood, bone, muscle and tendon health are so important for preventing osteoarthritis and for halting its progression. The body needs nutrition to be healthy.

Drinking too little water is also an issue because water keeps the tissue moist, the joints lubricated and the tendons and muscles supple. Dehydration does not allow the body to remove enough of the impurities and toxins that stress it. When these are left to recycle in the body, they can cause pain, swelling and inflammation making arthritis worse.

Exercise, like diet, is a two-edge sword. Too much can cause joint breakdown and too little can cause flaccid muscles which also cause joints to rub and break down cartilage. Too little stretching and rest also do not allow the body to repair itself and heal from the trauma placed on it by too much exercise. Too little exercise can cause arthritis symptoms to get worse, because by being immobile you lose flexibility, stability, range of motion and become stiff and painful.

If you do not focus on positive outcomes and take ownership of your arthritis, you will not be able to make powerful strides toward slowing the progression and reducing symptoms. Too little stake in your own health and making the necessary lifestyle changes is one of the detrimental downward spirals people get into once they are diagnosed with arthritis. Please don't allow yourself to be among them.

Arthritis Stagnations

When it comes to arthritis there needs to be a "moving along" of stagnations. Mainly these are experienced as tight, inflexible muscles that leave you unable to move freely. These cause trigger points, which lock toxins into the muscles, causing stiffness, pain and friction. When the body is in one place too long, like prolonged sitting or lying, it is stagnating in place. This is unhealthy, especially for arthritis, which needs a body moving to relieve symptoms.

Remaining in a holding pattern in terms of diet and nutrition is also a kind of stagnation. It means you have not made up your mind to eat right and take the supplementation necessary to help effect positive change. Don't stagnate when it comes to food, diet and supplementation. Make a change, even if it is a small change each week.

Your mind and emotions can also stagnate, or control you through their focus on the negative. Stress and anxiety make it hard to make decisions because you are worried of the outcome or afraid to begin a plan of change. Fear sets in and can be crippling. When you don't change your view on the subject of arthritis, your mind and emotions stagnate in the realm of the negative. This can create a negative worldview and halt (stagnate) change. Again, as with nutrition, you can make small daily changes in how you view your condition and can then create changes in behavior (and in your condition) over time. This can be hard at times, but it is vitally necessary.

Look at these two charts. The first, shows how the "Three Hidden Causes" are likely the "root" of your condition, and how they affect it. The second shows how the symptoms you experience are also related to excesses, deficiencies and stagnations.

ARTHRITIS "3 HIDDEN CAUSES" E.D.S. CHART			
	Excess	Deficiency	Stagnation
WEIGHT	Every 10 lbs over weight = 30 lbs extra compressive force on joints	Underweight = more nutrition needed to help repair and reverse arthritic damage	Remaining over or underweight pounds can worsen condition, prevent it from repairing and reversing
DIET	To much glucose, carbohydrates, inflammatory foods, diuretic beverages	Not enough water, thermogenic spices, anti-inflammatory foods, healthy fats and supplements	Unchanged diet = unchanged condition and contributes to worsening of symptoms
EXERCISE	Too vigorous, jumping and high impact = tough on joints	Sedentary, couch potato, unfit, atrophied muscles, loss of bone density	Buildup of lactic acid, muscle spasms, loss of flexibility
SLEEP	Over 8 hours daily can lead to lethargy, over tiredness, weakness, malaise and depression	Less than 8 hours daily = insufficient repair, lower production of serotonin, cramps, achyness and stiffness	Sleeping too long in poor posture can increase pain

ARTHRITIS "SYMPTOMS" E.D.S. CHART			
EMOTIONS	Stress, anxiety, worry, obsessing over your condition can lead to depression and feeling that nothing can be done.	Poor mental outlook can lead to unwillingness to help yourself, lack of dietary control, lazyness, loss of enthusiasm	Lack of passion for life, desires, loss of interest in things, activities and what life has to offer.
RANGE OF MOTION	Pain, inflammation caused by flacid ligaments, too much space between joints	Inability to move freely, bend joints fully, stand or walk without pain	Extreme limited movement causing frozen hips, knees, shoulder, fingers
PAIN AND INFLAMMATION	Reach for NSAIDs, muscle relaxers and invasive surgical procedures	Trigger points, muscle spasms, throbbing pain in fixed location	Doing nothing to help yourself, potential for endless suffering

RESTORING BALANCE IS THE KEY

It would be a mistake to assume that only one of these three causes is the root of any health condition. In fact, it is usually a combination of all three EDS that make a simple problem become chronic and seemingly complex. The first "cause" of an issue could be singular (i.e., an excess), but when not approached with the wellness model of health (i.e., restoring balance), it becomes multi-faceted.

The way to alleviate your arthritic condition and halt its progress is to consider it from this three-part perspective. If you can categorize where you are in excess you can then make changes toward decrease and balance. If you are able to list areas of deficiency you can then take steps to improve them. Where you find stagnations you can look for ways to "move them along."

Returning the body to homeostasis can be difficult and challenging. You may have been polluting your body with toxins in foods, beverages and air and aggravating it with stress, tension, poor sleep and bad lifestyle choices for quite some time.

In order to re-establish homeostasis – natural wellness balance – the many toxins and stressors that tax the body must be removed or, in the case of psychosomatic triggers, dealt with in new ways. This includes reducing food triggers, correcting musculoskeletal triggers, regulating biological functions, reducing the effects of stress and anxiety, keeping the body in a perpetual state of proper hydration and engaging in regular exercise.

A Dangerous Cycle

I hope you will find it easy to understand how these three EDS concepts – too much, too little and too slow – can contribute to and aggravate arthritis. It is important to know that they all happen at the same time. Consuming too much dairy means you are probably eating too little greens or consuming too little water. Too little exercise means you are sitting for too long. And the cycle of relationships continues in a spiral and of its own momentum. It is a dangerous and self reinforcing cycle.

To change that cycle, you need to make lifestyle changes and embrace methods of treatment that may seem out of the ordinary to you at this time. The goal is to restore balance in your life, body, thoughts and emotions and in your diet to create a positive change that can add years of quality to your life.

The Arthritis Action Plan entails lifestyle changes. Making such changes is the only way to correct imbalances and move toward an optimal state of health. In Section II, we'll look at the various modalities, diets and methods that are proven effective in treating and overcoming arthritis.

Chapter Review

- The secret to overcoming arthritis lies in understanding where it begins
- Three hidden imbalances derail your health and cause pain, illness, and arthritis symptoms
- Despite multiple types of arthritis and their myriad of causes, all are based in a combination of three types of imbalance, or hidden causes
- Restoring balance of Excesses, Deficiencies, and Stagnations is key to reversing arthritis
- You can prevent the symptoms of arthritis by correcting those imbalances through the Arthritis Relief Action Plan

SECTION II:

Natural Solutions Your Doctor Doesn't Know

CHAPTER 9

Avoiding the Pitfall of Wrong Arthritis Treatment

Since you are reading this book, I assume that you have arthritis and are looking for a better quality of life. I also assume that if you are at a point where you are turning to the pages of a stranger's book for help, you must have gone through your primary care physician and several specialists, and perhaps some alternative medicine options yet found no lasting relief or results. So perhaps you feel like nothing can be done or that your personal arthritis situation may be hopeless.

There is hope and I am certain more can be done for your condition than you imagine. Why do I think this? Because I have been where you are and I know how doctors and healers think. Therefore, I know the pitfalls of their methods and I can tell you how to avoid them.

The Common Pitfalls

As odd as it may sound, the reason many healthcare and wellness programs fail is a matter of education. More specifically, I am referring to too much education in one specialty field. You see, when a healthcare practitioner (in any field) goes from the broad understanding of the human body and illness pathology to a very narrow and specific field, it is like they strap on a set of horse blinders. You know, those dark leather things placed next to the eyes of horses that pull buggies in the street, so they don't get distracted by all the traffic. If you need a heart surgeon, then a specialist is what you want. For general health and wellness, you need a broader view and different perspectives because there usually is not a single root cause to your condition. Let me explain.

If you decide to remain in modern medicine, your options for treating arthritis are linked to drugs, rehab perhaps, injections (more drugs) and surgery. Why? Because modern medicine looks at the body as a biological system needing to be manipulated with drugs to hide its inherent warning signs that something is wrong (i.e., pain, inflammation). I mean, wouldn't you think it silly to just turn up the radio to block out the grinding sound your car engine may be making, rather than fixing the problem causing the sound? The sound is a symptom, and indicator, that something is worn with the vehicle. So masking out the sound with the radio (or taking drugs so you don't feel the pain), is not really a sound and lasting solution. What's more, they view the body as a mechanical system in need of some carpentry. Instead of sealing or restoring the cracked wood frame, they instead choose to knock it down and install a new one in its place. Museums and those with an aesthetic eye find value, beauty and function in the old.

I am not saying all of these methods of healthcare are not useful or even powerful. I am trying to get you to see how specialists can be blinded by their education as to other options and how sticking to one modality at the behest of the others may be keeping you in pain. This also holds true for alternative and holistic practices. For sake of argument and understanding, let's look at a few here.

If you see a chiropractor for your pain, they will diagnose and treat you from their perspective. In such a case, they view the spine as the central body part to adjust and keep free, supple and to keep the nerves that protrude from it free and unobstructed. After all, the nerves carry signals to and from the brain, so if they are impinged in some way through subluxation (vertebral misalignment) or muscle spasm (trigger point), they cannot transmit correct information. When this happens, the brain cannot send useful information back to the injured or ailed area. The problem is, not all types of arthritis or even body pain syndromes are related to the spine or can be corrected by releasing the impaired spinal nerves.

Acupuncture has a long and illustrious history as China's fabled and powerful healing system. It is based on the theories of meridian (energy) channels and the points of energy that fall along those channels. When the energy is stagnated, deficient or in excess (EDS), its normal flow is hampered and develops pain or disease (depending on blockage location). By inserting very thin stainless-steel needles into a selection of points, stagnations can be moved, deficiencies can be strengthened and excesses can be reduced. This leads to free-moving blood and energy in the body, thus promoting balance and pain free existence. However, not all health issues can be traced to an energetic root cause, though parts of them can be.

You see, while this method does indeed help people, they can only do so within the limits of their specialty, of the education and healing view of their practitioners. Have you experienced some of these treatments and found good results for a while and then they trailed off? If so, that is because the issues that the modality is best suited to treat have been corrected, leaving the "intractable" or difficult ones unchanged. Many arthritis sufferers are left less than enthusiastic with their results.

Everyone, whether doctor or healer, becomes so focused on the theories of their specific healing modality that they were unable to see the obvious. I saw it because I was looking at the theories of health from the opposite end of the spectrum. I was not only a student but also a patient who became a doctor to find a relief from the insider's perspective.

The Arthritis Relief Action Plan Works!

Remember my story about how I became a doctor of Oriental and alternative medicine to cure myself and found the answer? Here is the amazing part: *it was simple*. So very simple, I began to wonder why no one had discovered it before. And here's my explanation: It was a can't-see-the-forest-for-the-trees situation. It required a new way of thinking about illness.

My search was for a through-line, a single thread connecting all the various theories and modalities that could truly provide me (and later, my patients) with a lasting, proven, life-long way to cure myself. After a decade of trial and error and making left turns on the straight path to wellness, I developed what I passionately refer to as The Arthritis Relief Action Plan. It is, at last, a program for real change. I am pain and illness free because of it. You will be, too.

The essence is this:

- The Arthritis Relief Action Plan works, but *you* must commit to working it.
- To live in optimal health *you* must learn the essence of how health is derived and maintained.
- *You* must strive to have self-compassion.
- *You* must become the expert on *you* and your *individual* situation.

Before you move on please, once more, ask yourself these personal questions:

- Do you believe in yourself?
- Do you believe you can live a happy, healthy, pain-free life?
- Do you believe that once you understand the method you can affect your own self-cure?

I believe it and I believe in you. I know The Arthritis Action Plan works. And I know you can make it work, too. I also know you may think that nothing can be done for you. Yet here you are, reading this book. In your heart and brain you still hope that something can be done; you have not yet given up all hope. I know you believe that you will always have "to manage" your situation, "to live with" your ailment. Please believe me when I tell you, this is simply not the case.

You see, after I cured myself of my chronic headaches and musculoskeletal pain, I started working out the specifics of how to apply my personal method to hundreds of other health issues. As director of Integrated Energy Medicine, LLC, I gave over 3,000 treatments before moving out of private practice and into patient education, and achieved real and lasting success for my patients.

Right now, you have an idea as to *what* is wrong with your health, because a dozen physicians have labeled it. You just don't know *why* it is happening to you. You certainly know how much you want to feel great. You just don't know *how* to get there. The Arthritis Relief Action Plan is your map. You bring the *what* to the table, and I, as your guide, will tell you the *why* and show you the *how*. Together, we will bring the miracle of optimal health into your life.

To be at the point where you are psychologically ready to take control of your health takes great courage and discipline. Are you ready to stop playing the role of victim to ill health and passive follower of a physician or healer? I am confident you have what it takes to embrace The Arthritis Relief Action Plan and take back control of your life.

Here's to your new life of optimal health and pain-free living. And within the pages of the next chapters are the ways to make that happen.

Chapter Review

- The wrong approach to arthritis relief is a dead-end journey which you can avoid
- Avoiding the pitfalls of wrong treatment can improve your condition more than you can possibly imagine
- Many arthritis programs fail because they are too myopically focused, guided by specialists blinded by their education. You now understand t how sticking to one modality may be keeping you in pain
- Specialty methods can help people, but only with limits that aren't right for everyone
- The Arthritis Relief Action Plan helps you understand why you have pain, and what you can do about it

CHAPTER 10

Eating for Arthritis: Food for Pain, Inflammation and Weight Loss

Food is a critical piece of the wellness puzzle, especially when it comes to arthritis. In this condition, food can cause pain, inflammation and compressive force on the affected joints (through being overweight). The typical American diet supports ill health by consisting of an enormous amount of saturated and trans fat, sugar, processed meats, preservatives and a frightening amount of processed foods. However, a proper diet that is anti-inflammatory in nature and full of dense nutrients can reduce pain, inflammation and body mass to relieve those very symptoms. By switching to an anti-inflammatory diet consisting of healthy whole foods, you can actually decrease inflammation and ease the pain and discomfort associated with arthritis.

Foods That CAUSE Pain and Inflammation

When it comes to controlling inflammation, food is a double-edged sword that can both cause and reduce inflammation. There are dozens of foods that create inflammation in our bodies, and there are dozens of foods that reduce and/or prevent inflammation in our bodies. Consuming the right mix of these is essential to living a life with decreased arthritis symptoms. In times of injury or pain flare-ups, the foods you consume may be what keep the inflammation active well past its usefulness, and send your pain into chronic territory. This is unacceptable.

Here are seven categories of foods that should be avoided if pain and inflammation are a major symptom of your arthritis.

1. **Animal Milk Products**
   (Milk, Cream, Ice Cream, Cheese, Cottage Cheese, Yogurt)

2. **Hydrogenated oils**
   (Non-Dairy Creamer, Crackers, Cookies, Chips, Snack Bars)

3. **Nitrates**
   (Hot Dogs, Cold Cuts, Pepperoni, Sausage, Bacon, Liverwurst)

4. **Processed Sugars**
   (Candy, Soda, Bread, Bottled Fruit Juice, Cookies, Snack Bars)

5. **Nightshades**
   (Potatoes, Peppers, Tomatoes, Eggplant, Paprika)

6. **Convenience Foods**
   (French Fries, Onion Rings, Loaded Baked Potatoes, Fatty Burgers, Mexican Food, Pizza, Calzones, Stromboli)

7. **Processed White Flour Products**
   (Flour, Bread, Pasta, Pizza, Crackers, Pretzels, Donuts)

Are you surprised?

As you can see, most of the items on this list are actually the staple American diet. Is it any wonder Americans are among the most obese and pain suffering peoples in the world? If you look closely at this list, you will notice these ingredients are found in just about every snack, frozen dinner, bread and even so-called "healthy" foods. Whatever you do, don't believe the marketing. Read the labels instead.

Do yourself an easy, no-cost favor … stop eating foods from the above list if you have inflamed joints or are in pain. Merely eliminating these items from your diet will help stop the inflammation cycle when its natural course has been run. By eating these foods, you are increasing the longevity of the inflammation, and thus self-inducing your own chronic pain. Now that you know which foods actually cause inflammation or make it worse, let us look at those foods that can help reduce and even prevent inflammation.

Foods That Reduce Pain and Inflammation

We all know the food we eat is our primary source of nutrients and energy, and becomes the substance of our blood. In addition to oxygen and water, food is the substance of life. Food can make you strong and keep you in homeostatic balance. A diet high in fiber and whole foods, low in preservatives and unhealthy fat and infused with blood-invigorating aromatic spices can help reduce pain and inflammation.

It is essential to any healthful diet – especially a diet for arthritis – that you consume as much fresh, organic, whole foods as possible. Eating foods in or as close to their original state is one of the keys to being healthy, preventing self-induced diet-based inflammation and reducing the inflammation you are experiencing as a result of arthritis. Here is a list of the best foods known to prevent and help reduce inflammation and pain. These should be eaten throughout the day as part of balanced wholesome meals.

- Wild Alaskan salmon
- Fresh whole fruits
- Bright colored vegetables (*except nightshades)
- Green and white tea
- Purified and distilled water
- Healthy oils (olive, flax, hemp, safflower, hazelnut, coconut)
- Beef and poultry that is certified organic
- Nuts, legumes and seeds
- Dark green leafy vegetables
- Organic oatmeal (regular, not instant)
- Aromatic spices (turmeric, ginger, cloves, garlic, onion, coriander, ground mustard seed)

As you can see, a diet high in whole foods and low in preservatives and unhealthy fat is the key to an essential part of an arthritis relief plan. Not only do the above-listed foods actually work to reduce pain and inflammation, but support proper nerve function, muscle and bone health. Remember, the acid/alkaline or pH level of your body (which can cause or prevent inflammation), is related to the food you consume. Using this chart, see how what you consume on a daily or monthly basis may be contributing to the worsening of your arthritis.

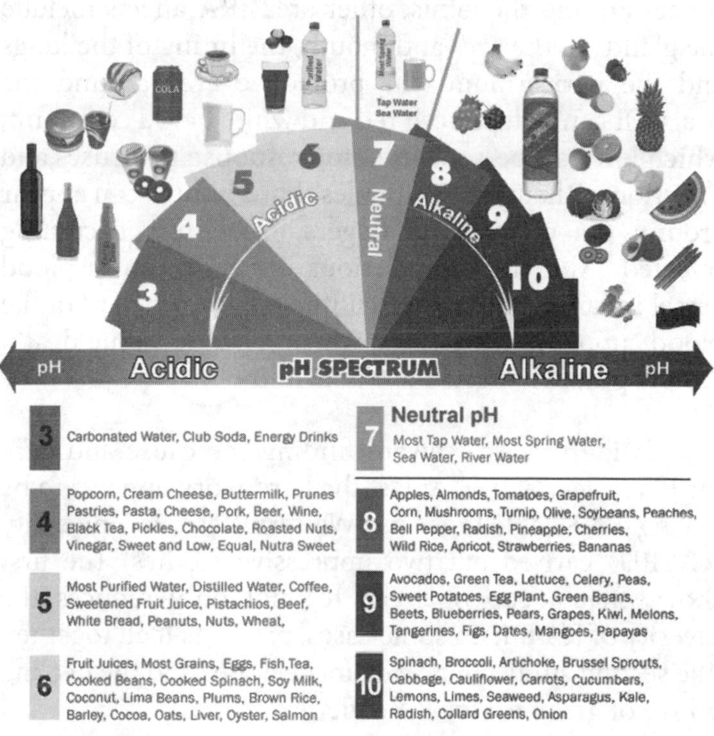

credit: mindbodygreen.com http://www.mindbodygreen.com/0-5165/Alkaline-Acidic-Foods-Chart-The-pH-Spectrum.html

Let's now look into a few of the super powerful consumables that are proven to relieve arthritis and the pain and inflammation associated with it.

Green Tea Reduces RA Symptoms

Each year, over two million Americans suffer excruciating pain from inflamed and swollen joints, crippled hands that can't hold a glass, even complete loss of some of their joints. The cause: Rheumatoid arthritis (RA). Besides the tissues around the joints, other areas RA affects include the glands of the eyes and mouth, the lining of the lungs and the pericardium (the protective area around the heart). It can reduce both red and white blood cell count, which lowers a person's immune response to viruses and infections. Rheumatoid nodules (hard lumps) can appear around the elbows and fingers, frequently becoming infected. And the most serious complication is blood vessel inflammation, or vasculitis, the impairment of the blood supply to the tissues, which leads to tissue death. Simply put, RA affects the whole body.

Worldwide research toward finding the cause and cure for RA is very active. At last the hard work appears to be paying off. Scientists at Case Western Reserve University (CWRU) carried out two impressive studies. The first shows that a cup of green tea not only reduces the severity of RA but, in some cases, prevents it all together. The second study offers even more hope as to the healing power of green tea for RA sufferers.

Green tea, like all true tea, comes from the leaves of the Camellia Sinensis tree, and 90 percent of the world's tea supply is produced in China. What makes green tea so powerful is a chemical compound called polyphenol, which occurs naturally in plants and works as an antioxidant. Polyphenols work to protect the body from the oxidative stress that causes diseases. Specifically, the polyphenol-Epigallocatechin Gallate (EGCG) is an extremely powerful antioxidant. In fact, EGCG antioxidant activity is more powerful than the antioxidants found in vitamins C and E.

After 15 years of working with green tea in his cancer research, Dr. Hasan Mukhtar started looking at the possible benefits this drink could have for people with RA. Realizing that both disorders were inflammatory in nature, his team began testing to see if green tea would have the same healing effect on RA as it does on cancer and cardiovascular disease.

His first paper, "Prevention of Collagen-Induced Arthritis in Mice by a Polyphenolic Fraction of Green Tea," was presented to the National Academy of Sciences in April 2005. The results were astounding. Out of the 18 mice that were given green tea extract, 10 never developed any arthritic symptoms and symptoms in the remaining eight had a much milder form of arthritis. The amount given was the equivalent of drinking ***Four Cups of Green Tea a Day!***

Lead author of the paper, Dr. Tariq M. Haqqi said, "Taken together, our studies suggest that a polyphenolic fraction from green tea that is rich in antioxidants may be useful in the prevention and onset and severity of arthritis."

Three independent and controlled experiments were conducted. Using a widely accepted animal model that is very similar to RA, the mice were injected with collagen to induce arthritis. Two groups were studied for 40 days, while a third was examined for 85 days to verify that the green tea did not simply delay the onset of the disease.

Green tea, unlike the more widely used black version, is not fermented. Instead of crushing the tea leaves, thereby removing the polyphenols, green tea is first dried, and then heated. One teaspoon steeped in hot (not boiling) water contains anywhere from 100 to 200mg of EGCG. Milk should not be added, as it negates the tea's beneficial properties. According to this study and others that were done for other diseases, two to four cups a day is usually recommended.

In a second study, researchers found further evidence that green tea is a powerful tool in the fight against RA. They discovered that the polyphenol ECGC could protect human articular chondrocytes from being destroyed in what is known as apoptosis, or cell suicide. These chondrocytes are cells that are responsible for releasing cartilage, the very thing that RA attacks. Dr. Haqqi said this exciting discovery, coupled with their earlier study, offers RA patients new hope. Though the existing damage RA may have caused will not be repaired, it seems green tea will aid in halting any further progress. And by sipping several cups of green tea every day, those who are genetically predisposed to RA may never have to suffer from its disastrous effects.

Human trials are currently being developed. In the meantime, however, Mukhtar and Haqqi both strongly encourage people to start drinking green tea. Nobody has shown any form of toxicity associated with tea, and with the tremendous amount of data showing its many beneficial qualities, it is a wise and wholesome preventive measure.

Mushrooms Boost Immunity, Offer RA Relief

Mushrooms should be a part of your daily diet, as they are full of nutrients and are power immune boosters. They are easily accessible in most markets and come in a variety of types and flavors, like shitake, maitaki, oyster, straw, reishi and others. The best part is that mushrooms are easy to grow at home. In fact, not much is needed to ensure a good crop, since they can grow in coffee grounds, peanut shells, cottonseed, cereal grain and even the pulp of citrus fruits. How easy is that?

There are six reasons mushrooms are so powerful and essential to health:

1. Mushrooms are an excellent dietary staple and health booster.
2. Mushrooms contain about 30 percent of high quality proteins and all nine of the essential amino acids we need.
3. Mushrooms' fat is unsaturated and in such low levels it's not really worth mentioning.
4. Mushrooms contain more mineral salts than most meat and nearly double most vegetables.
5. Mushrooms are high in phosphorus and potassium and also contain calcium,

magnesium, aluminum, zinc and copper, as well as vitamins B1, 2, 3 and 9.

6. Mushrooms are useful in the treatment of diseases caused by low immunity, such as rheumatoid arthritis, HIV, lupus, connective tissue disease, hypertension, heart disease, diabetes, kidney dysfunction, viral infections, malnourishment, cancers, tumors and convulsions.

With so much going for them, and all their amazing health benefits, what's not to love? So go ahead and give mushrooms a big welcome in your home. Add them to your meals where you can. You will feel a whole lot better because of it, especially if you suffer rheumatoid arthritis and osteoarthritis.

Turmeric: Nature's Powerful Anti-Inflammatory

In traditional cultures that are thousands of years old, like India, there are deep traditions of cooking daily meals with medicinal roots and herbs. These herbs act as preventive measures for sustaining good health, and prevention is the cornerstone of India's traditional Ayurvedic medicine. Turmeric is one such medicinal root that has made its way into a vast number of Indian recipes.

Aside from your standard chicken or goat curries, there is a whole list of Indian dishes that contain flavorful thermogenic ingredients like cardamom, coriander, ginger, cloves and turmeric. Not only are the recipes tasty, the ones containing turmeric are especially healthful because of its component called curcumin.

Research by Sarker et al. notes its powerful anti-inflammatory, anti-tumor and antioxidant properties. Moreover, the U.S. National Library of Medicine and the National Institutes of Health say: “Laboratory and animal research has demonstrated anti-inflammatory, antioxidant, and anti-cancer properties of turmeric and its constituent curcumin.”

Unlike aspirin or ibuprofen, turmeric’s curcumin reduces inflammation naturally, without damaging the liver or kidneys. It has been found especially helpful in treating conditions like arthritis, sports injuries, irritable bowel syndrome, Crohn’s disease, tendinitis and various autoimmune diseases. Some research even suggests that curcumin may also help those suffering asthma, inflammatory bowel disease and, yes, even cancer.

Since curcumin is an anti-inflammatory as well as an antioxidant, it is used for treating arthritis, wounds, digestive disorders, liver issues and in the prevention of cancer. It also helps reduce the side effects of chemotherapy. Statistics show that Asian children experience less incidence of leukemia than their Western counterparts, and a diet rich in turmeric may be the reason why.

Thousands of scientific articles on the efficacy of curcumin are found within the National Institutes of Health (NIH) Library of Medicine’s PubMed MEDLINE database. These show curcumin to be effective in the treatment of inflammation, wounds, cancer, heart disease and as a preventive measure against arthritis, Crohn’s disease, irritable bowel syndrome (IBS), neurological diseases, Alzheimer's disease, multiple sclerosis, type II diabetes, cataracts, cystic fibrosis, scleroderma and many others.

My advice is to include more turmeric in your diet. You can try to eat more Indian and Malaysian food or buy the ground powder and use it in your own cooking. If you don't find the flavor pleasing, you can purchase a high-quality curcumin supplement. In any case, make turmeric/curcumin part of your arthritic diet.

Water Hydrates and Flushes Toxins

It is vital that every human being drink ample amounts of water every day – especially those who suffer from pain conditions, like arthritis. Since water makes up roughly 75 percent or three-fourths of the human body (and 85 percent of the brain), it makes sense that no tissue, organ or gland can function properly without ample supply of this natural fluid. A sluggish digestive system, liver and kidneys contribute to and trigger pain processes. We humans would cease to exist without the magic elixir known as water, which, next to oxygen, is the most vital substance on Earth.

Drinking ample quantities of water every day is so important that for centuries many traditional cultures have used its healing qualities to cure and prevent various illnesses and diseases. Traditional Chinese medicine, for example, recognized the healing powers of water more than 3,000 years ago. Even Hippocrates, the father of modern medicine, was said to have drank and bathed in water to benefit from the healing properties of its mineral content.

Indeed, the mere consumption of this fluid can help restore the body to its natural state of homeostasis (balance) by clearing toxins, cleansing the colon, flushing the liver and kidneys and emptying the bowels. These are all necessary in the goal of becoming pain- and inflammation-free. The toxins trapped in muscle tissue (becoming trigger points) and accumulating in the joints as phlegm-rheum (hot, sticky fluids) create pain, redness, swelling and inflammation.

As the water content of tissues falls to a certain point because of dehydration, the bi-layer membranes that surround cells contract, forming a barrier that prevents further water loss. This obstructs the free movement of molecules, so metabolism and elimination are limited. Slow metabolism and elimination lead to build-up of toxins in the blood, which can manifest as chemically-induced headaches, fibromyalgia and the pain and inflammation associated with arthritis.

It is in part due to the overtaxing of the colonic track by overeating, ingesting foods high in nitrates and other chemical content, in addition to an abundance of sugars or alcohol, that one feels exhausted and lethargic, experiences seemingly unending dull headaches, catches colds easily or becomes seriously ill. It is precisely the absorption of the nutrients in the colon and intestines from the food we eat that prevents, causes or cures what ails us.

Research indicates that a thorough flushing of the mucus folds in the colonic tract where toxins and wastes generally remain will clean the system and keep the body healthy and the immune system strong – which is essential in preventing and treating RA. At the same time, quantities of water are known to revitalize the kidneys and liver. By drinking ample quantities of water, the colon will become more effective, thus increasing the quantity and supply of fresh blood that can then move throughout the body – reducing toxic buildup while increasing pain relief.

It is vital that every cell, tissue and organ in your body be sufficiently hydrated for your body to return to and maintain its natural state of homeostasis. It is only in this state that the chemical toxins that have built up in the body can be properly processed and eliminated. Water is the only substance that can properly hydrate the body; not caffeinated coffees and teas, carbonated sodas or sugar-filled fruit drinks. Only water, pure and simple as it is, will keep you healthy and help the body eliminate many of the underlying triggers affecting your health daily. So how much water is enough?

Much is written about the specific quantities of water needed for the body to function properly. Certainly, drinking a single glass of water at lunch or dinner will not do the job. While the FDA recommends six, eight-ounce glasses of water per day, others experts suggest consuming eight ounces of water per 20 pounds of body weight.

I personally go by what my body shows me in the color of my urine. When the urine stream is clear, I am properly hydrated. The more yellow it is, the more water my body needs. When urine is dark orange, you are in great need of liquids and it may take a day or two to replenish the water to a point where the urine is again clear. The caveat here is that certain supplements will change the color of your urine. So bear in mind, when taking supplements, that the first or second pass of urine afterward may be discolored. You should, therefore, space your supplements out (discussed later) to ensure a good gauge of hydration if you decide to use the "urine color" indicator, as opposed to drinking water based on weight.

Your body will never feel as light or as clean and unpolluted as it will once it is properly hydrated. And in the process, a large portion of the on-going headache triggers that have attacked you in the past will be eliminated.

Eating For Weight Loss

When it comes to food, forget diets. Really, it is all about balance. The important thing is to understand why food is necessary and then to know which foods promote wellness and which destroy it. Diets and the idea of diets are short-term eating plans for fast weight loss. These never work as they don't educate or help reframe the mind and emotions to change the eating patterns that perhaps caused the weight gain. When it comes to arthritis relief, losing weight is essential.

Recall the information in Chapter 2 on how compressive force on your arthritis joints is felt at a level three times your excess weight. For every 15 pounds you are overweight, your joints feel it as an additional 45 pounds. Relieving this is well within your control if you can get a clear picture of food and its role in weight gain.

On a basic level, food is fuel. It is part of the four life-sustaining elements we humans need to live (food, water, oxygen, sunlight). In terms of what the Chinese call qi or energy, food helps provide our bodies with life-force, or the energy for life. It nourishes the body, cells, organs, brain and every other tissue. Eating a better quality of food improves the quality of your life-force and produces a higher quality of life.

In the East, food is looked to for health, prevention of illness, and as medicine for relieving acute symptoms. Eating a healthful diet has been, until a recent invasion of Western fast food, a staple of Asian cuisine. In the United States, we think of food as a source of pleasure, social gathering and weight management. And that's problematic: We eat when we celebrate and when we're stressed, and we starve ourselves when we want to lose weight. This is an unhealthy attitude.

Trying to lose weight when you think of food as the enemy is unhealthy. You can't become thin and remain healthy when your diet restricts carbohydrates, protein, fruits, vegetables or other natural whole food sources. For weight loss to be healthy, your diet must encompass all that nature offers, in as close to its natural state as possible, or at least in an unprocessed state. Trying to lose weight by focusing on reducing calories or avoiding entire categories of food is futile. Just look at the thousands of past dieters who have tried this type of method and failed. Perhaps you are one of them.

When trying to eat for weight loss please keep these five points in mind:

1. Stop looking at each food in terms of its deconstructed parts, (i.e., its calorie, fat, protein and carbohydrate content). This tells only a

small part of the story and adds to confusion and stress.

2. Start looking at food in global terms of how an individual ingredient or product interacts with other food, and especially how your body handles it when eaten.

3. Remember that how much fat or carbohydrates a specific food contains on its own is not as relevant as what happens to it when it reaches your digestive tract. The important information is how quickly your body digests that food, how rapidly the food breaks down into sugar and how fast the food moves through the stomach and intestines. All of these depend on what else is consumed with it.

4. Forget about trying to lose weight with a diet and think instead of how to eat for optimal health, optimal energy and improved quality of life. Your weight will regress to the mean or reach an appropriate level based on your body and its needs.

5. Keep in mind that being skinny or thin has no relevance to being healthy. Skinny people also may have diabetes, heart disease, high cholesterol and other diseases related to diet. You should aim to be a healthy weight while fueling your body with nutrient-dense foods.

Along with the above five points, there are a few things I'd like to share that are the basis of healthful eating. Some of this may be familiar, and some may seem surprisingly counterintuitive.

Carbs

To begin, carbohydrates fuel your brain, so avoiding them as part of a diet will decrease your brainpower. Moreover, I cannot imagine anyone knowingly choosing decreased brain function as a matter of course to lose weight. It is a bad trade-off. However, you can choose to eat only complex carbohydrates like those from whole grain, fruit and vegetable sources. Whole grains take longer to break down and turn to sugar, meaning your body does not dump loads of insulin into your bloodstream at one time causing you to crash later and crave more simple carbohydrates. Simple carbohydrates are not healthy: They break down too quickly in your body, causing spikes in blood sugar, which causes weight gain from storing sugars and fats and indulging the consequent cravings.

Fats

Fats do not cause you to gain weight unless you eat them in abundance. In addition, the content of a fatty food tells only part of the story. For example, when you note the fat and cholesterol of bacon, you see numbers based on bacon in its raw state. Once the bacon is cooked, especially to crispy, a huge amount of its fat and cholesterol has been removed from the edible product.

Blood Sugar and Glycemic Load

More important than individual calorie and fat content of food is its glycemic load, or how quickly or slowly the body breaks down food, converts it to sugar and either uses it for fuel or stores it as fat.

A chart of glycemic loads lists each food based on its relative glycemic ratio of fiber to sugar content. The more a food is processed or has had sugar added, the higher its numerical index. In contrast, the higher its whole grain content, the lower its index number.

GLYCEMIC INDEX CHART

Low Glycemic (55 or Below) High Glycemic (70 or Higher)

SNACKS	G.I.	STARCH	G.I.	VEGETABLES	G.I.	FRUITS	G.I.	DAIRY	G.I.
Pizza	33	Bagel, Plain	33	Broccoli	10	Cherries	22	Yogurt, Plain	14
Chocolate Bar	49	White Rice	38	Pepper	10	Apple	38	Yogurt, Low Fat	14
Pound Cake	54	White Spaghetti	38	Lettuce	10	Orange	43	Whole Milk	30
Popcorn	55	Sweet Potato	44	Mushrooms	10	Grapes	46	Soy Milk	31
Energy Bar	58	White Bread	49	Onions	10	Kiwi	52	Skim Milk	32
Soda	72	Brown Rice	55	Green Peas	48	Banana	56	Chocolate Milk	35
Doughnut	76	Pancakes	67	Carrots	49	Pineapple	66	Yogurt, Fruit	36
Jelly Beans	80	Wheat Bread	80	Beets	64	Watermelon	72	Custard	43
Pretzels	83	Baked Potato	85	Onions	75	Dates	103	Ice Cream	60

Many individuals who struggle with weight do so because of problems with blood sugar, insulin resistance and metabolic issues that can be controlled by maintaining a glycemic load of 50 points or lower per day. In this way you fill your meals with food that breaks down slowly into sugars in your body and, therefore, does not promote too much insulin release and storage of sugars as fats.

Ideally, you want to break down your food slowly and use it as fuel as you go. Weight gain happens when the body stores unused food as fat or when too much insulin is released as a reaction to eating too many simple carbohydrates.

Look at the glycemic load chart above and consider how your daily eating habits are directly responsible for your weight issues, in addition to associated health issues like type 2 diabetes, metabolic syndrome and insulin resistance syndrome. If you eat whole foods and look to food as fuel for life-force, and not for weight loss, you can level off at a healthy weight by eating healthfully and not triggering an over-release of insulin from poor food choices.

Fat-Burning Foods for Weight Loss

When all is said and done, weight loss and the breakdown of food are linked to a properly working metabolism. That is, your body's process of converting food into fuel. Some people are naturally lean, and chances are they have a "fast metabolism." Other people just smell French fries and seem to put on weight; and they have what is called a "slow metabolism."

One of the secrets to weight loss and continued weight management, then, is to obtain and maintain a fast metabolism. The first step is to identify those things that slow down your metabolism.

There are five basic things that slow your metabolism:

1. **Low levels of physical activity** – Healthy weight loss depends on moving the body to increase heat to burn calories and invigorate digestion to break down food.

2. **The gradual loss of lean muscle tissue from that lack of exercise** – While muscle weighs more than fat, it is healthy and also helps burn fat. For healthy weight loss you must increase your muscle tone, and this can easily be done by walking with light hand weights and doing

simple chores about the house, like vacuuming and ironing, as long as you alternate hands. Activities like mowing the lawn and lifting weights are also helpful in this regard.

3. **Not eating regular well-balanced meals** – Every time you eat, your metabolism is jump-started. Food is fuel, and eating starts processes in motion in the body for breakdown, digestion and elimination. Not eating regularly sends your body into starvation mode, where it begins storing fat.

4. **Fasting or dieting that restricts caloric intake for extended periods** – This is unhealthy as it deprives the body of the essential nutrients it needs for optimal survival. Restricting calories depletes lean muscle tissue and when the diet is over people overeat in reaction to being "starved."

5. **Insufficient daily protein consumption** – Whether animal or plant as its source, it is advisable to consume protein every day. It gives your body energy and burns slower than carbohydrates, thus extending energy and stabilizing blood sugar levels.

Balancing the above five issues will help you turn a slow metabolism into a balanced, functioning metabolism. However, a normal metabolism is just the beginning and generally is insufficient on its own for many people's fat-burning goals. A fast metabolism, on the other hand, will help you reach and maintain an ideal weight and ratio of fat to muscle.

There are six basic ways you can improve your metabolism:

1. **Weight and strength training** will increase muscle tissue. The more muscle you have the more calories you burn throughout the day.

2. **Regular physical activity** will turn up the heat and melt the fat calories away. Regular fitness is best, but even small things like taking brisk walks, raking leaves and cleaning the house at a faster pace can burn more calories than taking an easier route.

3. **Keep hormones and blood sugar levels** stable by consuming whole grains (as replacement for processed simple carbs) and low-sugar foods while decreasing toxic preservative intake. Supplements can also help.

4. **Drink plenty of water** to keep the system working optimally. Water, pure and simple, can flush those toxins that make the metabolism sluggish.

5. **Eat smaller meals/snacks more often** by consuming a non-processed, healthy snack like a piece of fruit or nuts every three hours. By doing this, you will maintain a steady level of energy while also keeping your blood sugar levels from dropping. When blood sugar drops, unhealthy food cravings emerge.

6. **Eat foods that stoke your metabolism.** That's right, there are actually foods and spices that can stoke (rev up) your internal temperature, improve the breakdown of food and fat, remove

toxins and increase your metabolism. The list includes drinks, foods, spices and supplements.

Drinks

German researchers have proven that drinking 17 ounces of ice water daily can raise your metabolism by as much as 30 percent. This happens because it requires about 100 calories of energy to re-heat your body once it is cooled down. Just don't drink it with food, or the food will sit in your stomach while your body tries to re-heat itself.

On the other end is drinking hot green tea. The antioxidants in this tea will help eliminate toxins that cause metabolic sluggishness, and the drink itself has been shown in studies to increase metabolism.

Foods

Eating plenty of protein for energy and whole grain carbohydrates will do much to maintain energy, blood sugar levels and elimination schedules. The grains remove cholesterol from the blood and help maintain bowel function while the protein gives you sustained energy for exercise.

Spices

Some people complain that healthy foods do not taste good. To them, I say: Spice it up! Thermogenic spices, the heat-inducing aromatics, stoke the metabolism while making plain food taste great. These pungent spices heat up your body, causing it to sweat and burn fat. So include plenty of chilies, mustard, allspice, ginger, garlic, onion, curries, turmeric, cloves, cayenne and other aromatic spices to your diet and your metabolism will speed up by around 40 percent for roughly the next two hours.

So there you have it; ways to balance and boost your metabolism for weight loss and optimal health. Avoid the pitfalls that contribute to a sluggish metabolism while at the same time doing what you can to increase metabolic functions. There's never been a more tasty way to do it! And when it comes to reducing and preventing the negative side effects of arthritis, losing weight and keeping it off is an essential piece of the plan.

Chapter Review

- Food is a critical piece of the wellness puzzle, especially when it comes to arthritis
- Food can cause pain, inflammation and compressive force on the affected joints due to excess weight
- The typical American diet – filled with saturated and trans fat, sugars, preservatives, convenience food, and overly processed foods – is a deadly recipe for acidity, inflammation, and pain
- Avoid inflammatory foods and consume as much fresh, organic, whole foods as possible
- Eating a diet rich in anti-inflammatory foods, filled with dense nutrients, can reduce pain, inflammation and body mass
- Essential, yet often overlooked foods like green tea, mushrooms, turmeric and water, are proven to reduce inflammation and pain.
- When eating for weight loss, forget diets, forget counting carbs and calories. Stick to the basics of healthy eating. Stabilize your blood sugar by knowing the glycemic load of everything you eat and consume metabolism boosting foods and spices

CHAPTER 11

Natural Supplements for Arthritis Relief

This chapter begins by stressing the fact that natural supplements are not the same as chemically manufactured medicines. To begin with, they are made of natural ingredients and are less toxic and therefore less harmful to the body, if taken as directed. Even in low doses, many prescription and over-the-counter drugs are toxic and have short-term negative effects on the liver, kidney and digestive tract. When taken over the long term, or not as directed, the pharma meds can cause serious organ damage. Why?

Because drugs are created in a lab and our bodies are not equipped to digest and process them. Moreover, drugs are super powerful which gives them the ability to offer fast relief of symptoms, like pain and inflammation. This is good for short-term use, but can be harmful over time. The body just can't metabolize these drugs sufficiently to prevent them causing new damage and side effects.

Natural supplements, on the other hand, are made from the stuff of nature. This includes leaves, twigs, berries, bark, roots, vines, vitamins and minerals. They are natural substances that can't be regulated by the FDA because they are technically foodstuffs. If you understood herbology you could, as many traditional cultures do, adjust your diet to include the herbals in your meals. However, for painful and chronic conditions, like arthritis, this would mean at every meal. Taking these ingredients as supplements to your diet is the way to go.

In addition to the other methods and strategies discussed in this book, I recommend taking natural supplements that reduce pain and inflammation, protect joint health and promote healing without side effects. Below I offer an overview of 14 different supplements formulas or ingredients often found within such formulations. Read each, keeping in mind your specific condition and how some may be more effective for you than others.

Avocado Soybean Unsaponifiables (ASU)

ASU is a vegetable extract made from the oil of avocados and soybeans that is said to slow the progression of osteoarthritis. It slows down the production of inflammatory chemicals in the body and thus the breakdown of cartilage in the joints. It has also been found to spur new cartilage cell growth. It is available in capsule form at a recommended 300 mg daily.

Boswellia Serrata

Boswellia serrata is a traditional Indian Ayurvedic remedy for inflammatory conditions. It is extracted from the gum of the Indian boswellia tree and has been in use for centuries to treat joint pain and inflammation. It provides anti-inflammatory activity in areas where there is chronic inflammation by turning off the pro-inflammatory cytokines that begin the inflammatory process. Moreover, research shows that the acids contained within boswellia extract stop the formation of immune cells known as leukotrienes, which are responsible for inflammation. This then allows blood to flow unobstructed to the joints for healing and improved mobility.

Burdock Root

Burdock root is a natural botanical that is in wide use for many conditions, among them arthritic pain, swollen joints and rheumatism. More than anything else, clinical studies have found it most effective as a blood purifier that helps to rid the body of deleterious toxins and clear congestion from the circulatory, lymphatic, respiratory and urinary systems. Burdock is said to cleanse and eliminate long-term impurities from the blood very rapidly through its action on both the liver and kidneys. For those who suffer from arthritis and have taken too much Tylenol, burdock root has been clinical proven to protect the liver cells from the damage of taking acetaminophen. It is believed to stimulate the gallbladder and encourage liver cells to regenerate.

Cetyl Myristoleate (CMO)

Cetyl myristoleate (CMO) is a fatty acid, an ethylated esterified fatty acid derived from bovine tallow oil. Though it is similar to fish oil, it is made specifically to help joints through its action as a cellular lubricant. Clinical studies show CMO to be an effective anti-inflammatory compound that promotes healthy joint function. It increases joint flexibility and range of motion by lubricating the joint at a cellular level. It works to decrease inflammation specifically in the joints and lubricate their movement. In other words, it increases the fluids that cushion the space between the joint bones. CMO is reported to effect change at the cellular level, within the cell membranes themselves. It assists in the reduction and prevention of breakdown in joint cartilage. This can be especially helpful for those suffering degenerative osteoarthritis. The *Journal of Rheumatology* reported on a double-blind study of patients with chronic knee osteoarthritis where the CMO group saw significant improvement while the placebo group saw none. In fact, the scientists were so impressed with the results they concluded CMO "may be an alternative to the use of non-steroidal anti-inflammatory drugs for treatment of OA."

Chondroitin Sulfate

Within the cartilage around your joints is a chemical known as chondroitin. Chondroitin is naturally produced by the body. As you age, your natural supply starts to plummet. And a loss of chondroitin from cartilage is linked to a major cause of joint pain. Moreover, through wear and tear the joint cartilage breaks down, resulting in the condition of Osteoarthritis. We can't regenerate cartilage on our own, but we can take a supplement called chondroitin sulfate which, studies show, can help slow down this degenerative process and help reduce arthritic pain. Chondroitin sulfate is made from the cartilage of cows and other animals, and is often used in combination with other products including glucosamine and manganese.

Citrus Bioflavonoids

Sometimes referred to as vitamin P, citrus bioflavonoids enhance the absorption of vitamin C and act as important antioxidants. Flavonoids also inhibit collagenase and elastase, the enzymes responsible for the breakdown of connective tissue. Connective tissue breakdown is one of the factors that may cause arthritis. Flavonoids reinforce the natural structure of collagen, improve the integrity of connective tissue, and protect against free radical damage.

Devil's Claw

Direct from the Kalahari Desert comes devil's claw, a claw-shaped fruit that has been used for centuries by the South African tribes to treat arthritis pain. Numerous studies carried out on devil's claw show it to have powerful natural NSAID-like properties. In fact, the journal *Phytomedicine* reported that it is just as effective as the osteoarthritis medication Diacerein. What's more, studies carried out in both France and Germany pointed to devil claw's effects being similar to cortisone.

Fish Oil / Omega-3 Fatty Acids

The omega-3 fatty acids found in abundance in fish oil derived from cod, trout, herring, salmon and other cold-water fish are proven to reduce inflammation. Research from Cardiff University in Great Britain found that cod liver oil not only relieves pain, but also stops and even reverses the damage caused by osteoarthritis and rheumatoid arthritis. Omega-3s help morning stiffness, regenerate joint tissue and have been shown to also aid in autoimmune disease like RA, lupus and psoriasis.

According to recommendations of the Arthritis Foundation, when treating conditions related to arthritis it is best to use "fish oil capsules with at least 30 percent EPA/ DHA, the active ingredients. For lupus and psoriasis, 2 grams EPA/DHA three times a day. For Raynaud's phenomenon, 1 grams four times a day. For rheumatoid arthritis, up to 2.6 grams fish oil (1.6 grams EPA) twice a day."

Glucosamine Sulfate

Glucosamine is one of the most-studied supplements around the world for relief of arthritis symptoms and joint health. Sulfur is produced naturally in the body and is an essential component to joint health. Glucosamine sulfate is a type of glucosamine that is most useful in the support of joint mobility and pain relief because it absorbs well. Conversely, glucosamine chondroitin does not absorb in an amount significant enough to create enough of a change to make taking it worthwhile. Glucosamine sulfate works as well as NSAIDs for some people but without the negative effects to the gastrointestinal tract or liver.

Hydrolyzed Collagen Type II

Collagen – particularly Type II collagen – is the main structural building block of joint cartilage. The human body is made up of 60 percent Type II collagen, and Hydrolyzed Type II collagen contains the amino acids found in human cartilage. Your body uses these amino acids to create new collagen – and repair your cartilage and connective tissue throughout your body. Hydrolyzed Collagen Type II also contains Hyaluronic Acid, which lubricates your joints.

Ionic Minerals

The human body is a miracle of electrical impulses that keep it functioning and make life possible. Ionic minerals are an essential part in this process, as the body relies on them to conduct and generate electrical impulses. Without the correct balance on ionic minerals in the body, your brain and muscles could not function properly and cells could not properly absorb nutrients.

There are over 70 trace minerals that are important to cellular, neurologic, joint and bone health. Taken together, ionic minerals balance and replace electrolytes, maintain pH balance, improve circulatory health and aid absorption of vitamins and nutrients.

Since most people do not live by the sea and much of our soil is depleted of minerals, many are deficient in these essential elements. Taking supplements containing ionic minerals can help arthritis in many ways, as long as the minerals are produced in water soluble form. A few of the most important ionic minerals are:

Boron helps metabolize calcium and magnesium and is critical for healthy membrane function.

Calcium is important for healthy teeth and bones and helps regulate nerve function.

Copper is essential for healthy function of proteins and enzymes and aids in the absorption of iron.

Iron is needed to transport oxygen to the cells in your body.

Magnesium helps relax muscles and stimulate enzyme production, in addition to regulating bowl function to help eliminate toxins.

Manganese promotes healthy bone formation, supports growth of healthy connective tissue and boosts calcium absorption.

Phosphorous helps repair damaged cells and promotes healthy new cell growth.

Selenium is a powerful antioxidant that helps vitamin E protect cells and connective tissue by destroying free radicals.

Zinc helps boost white blood cell production in your immune system.

L-glutathione

Glutathione is a natural protein found within every cell in the body and consists of the amino acids Glutamic acid, L-cysteine, L-glycine. It is produced by the liver and is also found in fruit, vegetables and meats like mutton, lamb and beef. It is the most powerful antioxidant in the body and helps protect cells from free radical damage and oxidative stress, thereby improving cellular health and strengthening the immune system. As such, in addition to a host of other diseases, L-glutathione is useful in the treatment of rheumatoid arthritis.

Methylsulfonlylmethane (MSM)

MSM is a potent sulfur naturally found in plants, animals and humans that helps rebuild the connective tissue in your joints. What's more, MSM has the unique ability to improve cell permeability. This allows harmful toxins to flow out, while allowing health boosting nutrients to flow in to feed your joints, cartilage and connective tissue. It is used for hundreds of symptoms related to a myriad of health diseases and conditions, and is especially effective at relieving inflammation for improved joint function, and pain associated with joint inflammation, osteoarthritis, rheumatoid arthritis, osteoporosis and tendonitis. One study published in the *Journal of Anti-Aging Medicine* found that MSM provides an 80 percent greater reduction in pain compared to the placebo.

Paractin

Paractin is a clinically proven extract of the medicinal herb Andrographis Paniculata, which helps correct an imbalanced immune system. This helps cut off the signals that cause inflammation and significantly decrease joint pain, which makes it a great ingredient in supplements for arthritis.

Proteolytic Enzymes

For arthritis relief, it is important to have proteolytic activity on the systemic level. Known as protease, this category of enzymes acts as a catalyst in the breakdown of proteins into peptides or amino acids. This helps control both systemic inflammation and inflammation resulting from soft tissue injuries, like those associated with both rheumatoid and osteoarthritis. Proteolytic enzymes also provide essential antioxidant and cardiovascular support. I will discuss two of the more potent ones here:

Bromelian is a mix of proteolytic enzymes (those found in pineapples), which have been used for centuries to help indigestion and reduce inflammation. Studies indicate this product helps reduce pain associated with arthritis, especially when used in combination with some other natural pain-relieving agents.

Papain contains a wide array of proteolytic enzymes, incorporating a broad range of substrate specificity and optimum environments. Because of this attribute, Papain easily and efficiently hydrolyzes most soluble protein, yielding peptides and amino acids. Papain has an effective pH range of 3.0 to 10.5.

Rutin

Rutin is a flavonoid composed of the flavonol quercetin and the disaccharide rutinose. Rutin is found naturally in a variety of plants, and dietary sources include black tea and apple peels. Rutin's anti-inflammatory potential is attributed mainly to its powerful antioxidant activity. Rutin also helps maintain the levels of reduced glutathione, which is a powerful biological antioxidant. The combination of these activities helps to minimize the cellular damage and resulting inflammation caused by the various oxidative processes.

SAMe (S-Adenosyl methionine)

SAMe is one of the natural chemicals made within the body that science has been able to duplicate in a lab, and make into a supplement. Studies have shown SAMe supplementation to be comparable to the pain-relieving effects of Celebrex by the second month of taking the product, without the side effects. The SAMe chemical has a role in pain, depression, liver disease and has been shown effective when used for relieving the symptoms of osteoarthritis, fibromyalgia, bursitis, Alzheimer's disease, multiple sclerosis (MS), migraine headache, depression and more.

Thunder God Vine

China, Korea and Japan grow a vine known as Thunder God, which is one of the powerful natural relievers of arthritis, especially RA. It has properties that regulate the immune system and reduce inflammation, thus being good for autoimmune diseases. One clinical trial carried out at the University of Texas Southwestern Medical Center discovered that roughly 80 percent of those patients who were given a high dose of the plant supplement found that their rheumatoid arthritis symptoms got better considerably.

White Willow Bark

Since the time of Hippocrates white willow bark has been in use as a natural means of reducing inflammation and pain, specifically associated with osteoarthritis and rheumatoid arthritis, as well as headache, backache, gout and PMS. The bark of the willow tree contains the chemical salicin, which has a similar effect in the body as acetylsalicylic acid (aspirin). But it's better than aspirin, because it has none of the gastrointestinal side effects, and it naturally contains flavonoids (anti-inflammatory compounds found in plants).

Vitamins

Vitamins are essential to health. Every natural thing that you eat contains the vitamins needed for growth, repair, bone density, pH balance and hormone regulation. The problem is that many people don't have access to organic whole foods, so vitamin supplementation is important. When suffering from arthritis, the following vitamins may help.

Vitamin B12 is a nutrient that promotes healthy blood cells, prevents anemia and fights off inflammation of the joints and helps make DNA. It is essential for the normal functioning of the cells, nervous system and gastrointestinal tract.

Vitamin D3 is a fat soluble vitamin that promotes calcium absorption and enables normal mineralization and growth of the bones. Deficiency of Vitamin D3 (the active source of Vitamin D) can lead to loss of bone density, brittle bones or misshapen bones. Ample levels can help prevent osteoporosis. It is important that you ask your healthcare provider to test your Vitamin D blood levels, to ensure you do not get too much.

Vitamin E is a fat-soluble and essential nutrient for humans. The most important components of vitamin E appear to be the tocopherols. All four forms of tocopherol have been shown to have antioxidant activity, but alpha-tocopherol is the strongest antioxidant. Alpha-tocopherol inhibits the oxidation of LDL, which can help prevent LDL from sticking to the arterial walls. In addition to its antioxidant properties, vitamin E also acts to reduce blood coagulation and may help to lower blood pressure by eliciting endothelial relaxation.

Vitamin K2 helps prevent osteoporosis by keeping calcium in your bones where it belongs. Without vitamin K2, calcium floats through your bloodstream and sticks to places it doesn't belong, like your blood vessels.

How to Take Natural Supplements

Because natural supplements are made of organically existing substances, they affect the body in gentle ways - without side effects. The ingredients within natural supplements often do not work as quickly as drugs do at relieving pain or inflammation. However, they do offer acute relief in the short term while working more powerfully over time to create a gradual and lasting change in condition. In other words, supplements need to build up in your system to get to a level where more significant change occurs, which is why you often will need to take them several times per day, over periods of weeks and months or even longer.

The best way to take supplements is by following the guidelines on the label. These guidelines are often the minimal doses and therefore for acute conditions the doses can be increased, sometimes doubled or tripled. However, in high doses even natural substances can become toxic in the body. In all cases, it is necessary to use caution and to take supplements and medications as directed on the bottle or as suggested by a professional healthcare provider.

Note: For information on the arthritis herbal formulas used in traditional Chinese medicine (TCM), please refer to the Appendix. Because these products are less available to many, and require an exam by a licensed TCM practitioner before use, they have been moved to an Appendix.

Chapter Review

- Natural supplements are far superior to chemically manufactured medicines
- When taken as directed, natural ingredients in supplements are less toxic to the body, and can reduce pain and inflammation, protect joint health, and promote healing without side effects
- Natural supplements affect the body in gentle ways, and therefore require more time to build up in the body and make a positive change
- Certain supplements provide vitamins and minerals that are difficult or nearly impossible for us to get naturally, yet understanding the source of them is crucial to health
- Supplements with some of the following ingredients are critical to relieve pain and inflammation associated with arthritis: Biofermented Hyaluronic Acid, Chondroitin Sulfate, Omega-3 Fatty Acids, Glucosamine Sulfate, Methylsulfonlylmethane (MSM), Proteolytic Enzymes, SAM-e, Water-Soluble Trace Minerals, White Willow Bark
- When taking supplements, always follow the guidelines on the label and discuss with your health care provider

CHAPTER 12

Topical Creams, Gels and Oils for Arthritis Relief

When searching for relief from pain, inflammation, swelling and stiffness, many reach for some form of topical cream, gel or ointment. These products are found in abundance in American drugstores and in Asian markets. Though the Eastern and Western versions of these products have some different ingredients, they serve the same purpose: instant relief for acute symptoms of arthritis.

Topical pain products are mostly used for short-term relief, as once their active ingredients have metabolized in the body, their value is greatly diminished. For effectiveness over the long term they should be applied three times per day, and be part of an overall program for arthritis relief. On their own, these products can provide almost instant relief on some level to one or more symptoms and can be used to help you get through your day or night.

I use topical products when I am in too much pain to stretch or exercise, to help stimulate blood flow, reduce inflammation and curb the pain that would otherwise keep me from doing so. If you are not using these products, I suggest that you do. If you are unsure which product to try out – and it may take trying several for a week or so to find the best one for you – this chapter aims to give you the scoop.

How Topical Products Work

There are several key ways in which the various topical products help reduce pain, swelling, inflammation and stiffness. Many of the products are known as counter-irritants. This is a fancy way of saying they irritate your skin in some way to shift your mind and nervous system off the pressing issue. In other words, ingredients like menthol, wintergreen oil and eucalyptus are used to counter the symptomatic irritant by creating a new irritant, like redness or sensations of cool or warmth on the skin.

This process is also known as "gate control" or "gating," as it gates off or blocks the receptors in the skin from sending pain signals to the brain, instead sending the heat or cooling signal. This then "tricks" the mind to focus on the new irritant, and tricks the nervous system into think the area is hot (to send more blood) or cold (to send more heat) and, thus, improve the bothersome symptoms.

Many of the topical products contain salicylates, which is a class of chemicals that acts in a way similar to NSAIDs. In other words, they have topical analgesic (pain reducing) and anti-inflammatory (inflammation reducing) qualities. These chemicals appear in nature in mint, menthol and peppermint, for example. They work by inhibiting the synthesis of prostaglandin, the naturally occurring and chemically related fatty acids that aid in blood pressure and body temperature regulation and control inflammation and vascular permeability. Like NSAIDs, they can be useful in reducing fever, pain and inflammation in arthritis.

A Look at the Common Ingredients

Many of the most popular pain-relieving creams and gels share common ingredients. If you look at the product labels, you will likely see one or more of the following active ingredients, among others: wintergreen, camphor, menthol, capsaicin and salicylate.

I don't recommend using topical products that contain only one active ingredient because they don't address enough of the arthritis symptoms. I also do not recommend products that contain synthetic or chemical ingredients. For our purposes, please choose to use only those products containing all-natural ingredients.

First, the purpose of this chapter is to suggest that you try these several times per day as part of the overall program to overcome arthritis. Secondly, it is to educate you to know enough to make better choices when it comes to decisions about treating your arthritis symptoms. Let's now look at the common active ingredients in more detail so you can see which may be more useful for your condition.

Camphor Oil

Camphor oil, which is extracted from two types of camphor trees, also has many healthful properties that help alleviate the symptoms of arthritis. Most notably, it is a stimulant, calms nerve pain, reduces inflammation and is used as an anaesthetic, disinfectant and sedative.

While camphor has a cooling affect on the area it is applied to, it stimulates blood flow, helps metabolism and causes sweating of fluids, especially in and around the joints, to reduce swelling. Its cooling nature makes it a great anti-inflammatory agent. It is very useful at reducing pain through its temporary numbing of the sensory nerves and its vasoconstriction (blood vessel contraction), which takes pressure off swelling around nerves. It also has the ability to reduce the nervousness associated with pain and arthritis.

Please note that while an effective topical agent, camphor oil is a toxic substance that can be fatal if ingested (as little as 2 grams). **External use only**.

Capsaicin

Chili peppers are not just for eating anymore. Well, parts of them anyway. Capsaicin is the compound that gives the chili its heat and pungency and is the aspect that helps with the symptoms of arthritis. While the heat feeling of capsaicin may feel harsh at first, it does lessen with time. After a few weeks, you may not feel the same "heat" feeling, yet the healing effects continue. Capsaicin is found in topical patches and pain creams.

Like the other active ingredients of topical products, capsaicin is a counterirritant that produces a hot, burning sensation on the skin where applied. This tricks the brain into thinking the area is hot and it sends blood there, which helps with stiffness and pain and hyperactive nerve firing. Capsaicin also works by diminishing the chemical in the body known as substance P, which is involved in transmitting pain signals to the brain.

Menthol

Not only is menthol a popular pain reliever, it is also found in thousands of popular products, including mouthwash, toothpaste, breath mints, lip balm and pain-relieving creams. An organic compound derived from the mentha (mint, peppermint) family of plants, menthol is one of nature's best analgesics, for three reasons.

First, when menthol is included in a delivery agent, like topical gels and creams, molecules called ligands attach themselves to receptors in your cells, triggering a change. The menthol ligand attaches to the kappa opioid receptor, which produces a numbing effect.

Second, menthol triggers vasodilation or the expanding of blood vessels. This increase expands the blood vessel and thus increases the flow of blood to the area. As this happens the skin (barrier) is compromised in a good way, allowing other active and inactive ingredients found within the menthol product to penetrate the skin and affect the muscle soreness, joint stiffness and pain.

Third, menthol is an antipyretic, meaning it has a natural cooling effect on the body area in which it is applied.

It is one of the anti-irritants in that it fools the nervous system into thinking the body is cold, leading the nerves to send back a signal to relieve the heat of inflammation.

Wintergreen

The oil made from wintergreen leaf is often applied locally at the site of pain for treatment of arthritis, rheumatism, lower back pain, sciatica, headache, menstrual cramps and for pain and swelling and fever and nausea.

In high concentrations wintergreen acts as a rubefacient, which is another way of saying it is a counterirritant. Specifically, though, rubefacients cause redness of the skin by dilating blood capillaries, thus increasing blood circulation to the area where the product was applied. Once wintergreen is absorbed into the skin and metabolized by the body, it changes into a salicylate and therefore acts like an NSAID. If you have allergies to aspirin or salicylates, do not use products containing wintergreen oil. If not, give them a try.

Best Way to Use Topical Products

This piece of advice may sound silly, but here it is: Please read the labels of any of the products you are going to use prior to applying to your body. Many are harmful if applied to open wounds and scratches, if they touch the eyes or are accidentally ingested. Make sure you know the possible negative effects and have a plan for washing the affected area or otherwise in case of ingestion, etc.

Aside from that, these are simple to apply whether they are in cream, lotion, gel or salve form. Simply place some on your fingers and massage into the affected area. Where there is more bone, like the fingers, use gentler strokes and work in the product over time. Where there is more muscle, like the lower back or above the knees, you can press more deeply and massage the area while applying the product.

These products are made more powerful (or at least felt more) when applied right before or after a workout or hot shower, as the skin pores and blood vessels are expanded and can absorb more product more quickly. However, be warned that this may be too much to handle. If the product brings a heat sensation, it will be increased many fold and may be unbearable. Also, be sure to wash your hands immediately after application to prevent accidental touching of your eyes, face, mouth or private areas.

Part of maintaining an effective wellness program, like the overcoming arthritis program presented in this book, is to have realistic expectations of what may happen. Keep in mind that while effective at reducing acute symptoms like pain and inflammation, topical products often take around two months to have longer lasting effects. You should look to them as products to support symptomatic relief in the moment, and will eventually have longer-lasting relief. In any case, they should be used as a supportive part of a broader program of relief and this is how they are viewed within this program.

Note: For information on the topical arthritis products used in traditional Chinese medicine (TCM), please refer to the Appendix.

Chapter Review

- Topical products can produce short-term improvement; longer-term effectiveness requires application three times per day
- Look for topical products with salicylates, which relieve inflammation and reduce pain, similar to NSAIDs, but without the negative side effects
- Popular pain-relieving creams include wintergreen, camphor, menthol, capsaicin, and salicylate in their ingredients
- For best results, topical products should also contain ingredients found in supplements such as: Hyaluronic Acid, MSM, Chondroitin Sulfate, Glucosamine Sulfate, L-glutathione, White Willow Bark, and others
- Avoid using topical products that contain synthetic or chemical ingredients

CHAPTER 13

Ancient Exercises for Arthritis Relief

I am often asked what type of exercise program one should begin as part of a program for arthritis relief. There are so many different types of exercises available and so many places to do them, that to begin such a program can seem daunting, especially if a sedentary lifestyle has been the norm. If you add to this a condition like arthritis, where there is a constant degree of stiffness, inflammation, swelling and pain in the joints and surrounding muscles and tissues, picking the *correct* program is essential. After all, while exercise is a vital part of overcoming arthritis, the wrong kind of exercise can make the condition worse overall.

When considering exercises for arthritis, they must do the following:

- **Promote Circulation**
- **Relaxed Contracted Muscles**
- **Tone Flaccid Muscles**
- **Increased Range of Motion**
- **NOT Stress the Joints**
- **Not Aggravate the Arthritic Condition**

There is also the mental and emotional component to consider. Engaging in an exercise program that is or seems daunting may be overwhelming and cause you to quit too soon or not begin at all. Any health approach should incorporate an integrated mind/body theme. This is an essential component of the physical activity you choose as exercise. In addition to burning calories, increasing oxygen intake, stabilizing blood fats and sugars and releasing those feel-good hormones, you will also develop a mind/body center that will help focus your thoughts, emotions and spirit, thus helping to reduce the stress and anxiety that often accompany arthritis.

I would like to share four exercise methods that are aligned with the components mentioned above, and are enjoyable and easy to do. They will get you toned and help you lose weight while also connecting your mind and body. These are Mindful Walking, QiGong Standing Pole, Wu Style Tai Chi and Yoga.

Mindful Walking

Exercise (even in small doses) is necessary to reduce the symptoms of arthritis because it gets everything moving: the heart, the lungs, the muscles and the joints. To start feeling relief, get your body moving for 20 minutes per day. Even low-impact walking is enough movement to help stop the pain-pill-inactivity-pain cycle.

Walking is an aerobic activity, but since it is low-impact there is little wear and tear on the joints and little (if any) triggering of pain from the jarring action of the body — as experienced in high-impact aerobic exercise or jogging. Although it is a simple activity, walking actually utilizes most of the muscles of the body to propel you forward and keep you in balance while increasing respiration, heart and lung function, blood and oxygen flow, the "burning off " of blood sugars and fats and removal of toxins and other wastes through sweat and improved eliminative functions. All of this, of course, causes a vast decrease in pain.

Walking is so simple and *ordinary*, yet in one 20-minute session you can raise HDL (good cholesterol levels), increase respiration within safe limits, sweat out toxins, release the endorphin feel-good hormones, improve heart function, begin reducing weight, reduce stress, promote relaxation and improve overall endurance and body tone. Amazing!

Many of the triggers that attack your health and cause pain can be reduced or eliminated simply by walking. And this activity only requires time, as no special place need be made to do it — although it is preferable to walk in a park as opposed to a busy city sidewalk.

Though walking in and of itself is a common activity, few of us do it properly. In fact, walking as we naturally do offers little for the purposes of overcoming arthritis. You must look to walking as a mind/body activity, wherein your mind is clear, emotions calm, respiration steady, body properly aligned and relaxed with each walking step even and balanced. If you are able to integrate each of these components while walking for at least 20 minutes a day, then your walks can be considered a microcosm of an integrated mind/body approach to health and wellness … and you will begin to derail the chronic pain cycle on your first outing.

QiGong Standing Pole Exercises

QiGong energy work is now quite popular in the West. Yet for centuries it has been a part of the Eastern way of life. In China, people can be found in droves in the local parks at the break of dawn practicing QiGong and Tai Chi to maintain or regain their health. QiGong are systems of concurrently exercising the body and the internal organs to stretch the body, open the meridians (energy lines), release tension, clear the mind, balance respiration and improve the circulation of energy, blood and body fluids. All of this is achieved in relatively brief exercise sets that are simple and effective against pain, stiffness and disease.

Regular practice of QiGong exercises aid in regulating the functions of the central nervous system. Along with exercising and controlling one's mind and body, QiGong influences one's physical states and pathological conditions. There are both practitioner applied and individual self-regulating QiGong methods. In this chapter we discuss the self-regulating practices.

While there are literally hundreds of different QiGong practices, they all have a similar theme and purpose. I will describe the method known as *zhan zhuang*, or simply the "standing pole" method. It requires only enough space to stand still, and it is so simple that you will not be distracted by having to remember specific sequences of movement.

This practice is easy. Stand with your legs shoulder-width apart, knees bent only one to two-inches, with both arms bent and held at the same level. Below are three standing postures for you to do in sequence.

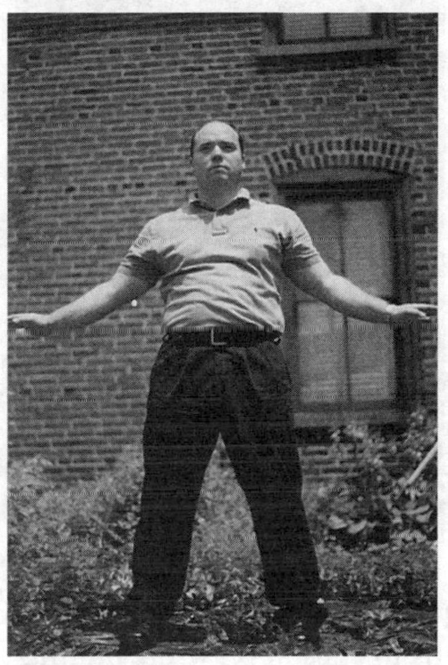

1 – Hand Floating on Water. Hold your arms out to their sides, palms facing down. Visualize that your palms are floating on water. Be sure to keep them in place and not move them during the exercise.

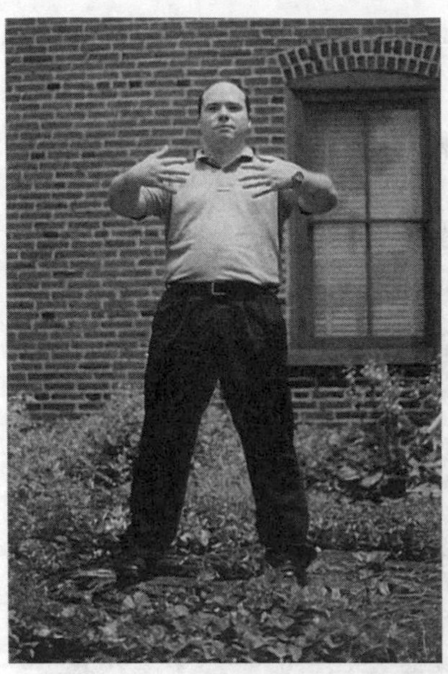

2 – Hugging a Tree. From the previous posture, slowly raise your arms to chest level while pulling them slightly inward. You want to feel as if you are hugging a tree, which is a mental image to keep your arms from coming too close to the body. Relax your hands, elbows and wrists, again like they are floating on water.

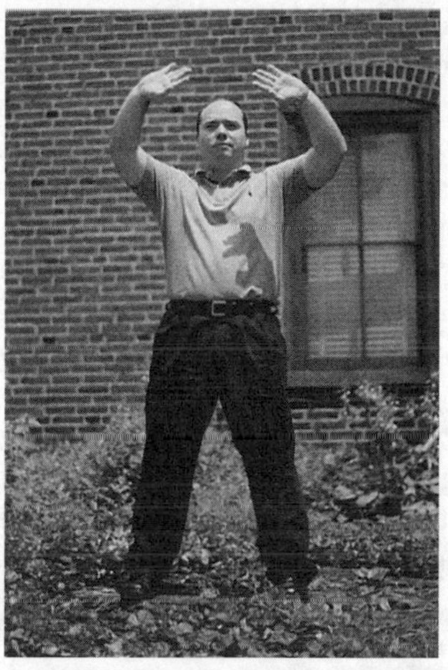

3 – Holding Up the Sky. From the previous posture, slowly rotate your palms outward while lifting your arms upward. The final position should find your hands at about forehead height, extended slightly forward and upward, as if holding up the sky from falling.

Once the posture is assumed, do the following three steps:

1. **Quiet Your Mind** by not stressing over distracting thoughts that may come – simply allow them to go freely without passing judgment.

2. **Regulate Your Respiration** by quietly breathing in and out at a steady relaxed pace. Continue doing this and enjoy yourself for the next nine minutes.

3. **Transition** to the next posture. After nine minutes, slowly move your arm position to the next posture. Do not excite your mind or move your legs, as this will distract your energy and intention.

This sounds so simple yet there is quite a bit going on as explained in a quote from *Traditional Chinese Therapeutic Exercises – Standing Pole,* by Wang Xuanjei and J.P.C. Moffett:

> "Standing pole is an exercise of the whole body. As the outer form of the body is not moved, all the internal organs settle, while all metabolic functions increase. This develops movement within non-movement, that is, unhindered internal activity and movement within external stillness. It is a non-violent and non-overburdening exercise, simultaneously providing rest and exercise, easily adaptable to any condition and encouraging development of the body's innate strengths and abilities in a natural way."

You see, although it appears as if you are doing nothing, the body is really engaged in a process of physical activity. While quieting the mind and regulating respiration you are reducing stress, relaxing the cerebral cortex and rejuvenating the central nervous system. You are also working muscles by virtue of maintaining an isometric posture wherein the knees and elbows are bent, the arms are raised and this must be held steady without release until the end of the session. This elevates heart rate without overtaxing the heart, improves the circulation of blood and oxygen throughout the body and increases metabolic functions while releasing toxins and tension from the body.

QiGong standing pole postures are a great way to begin exercising the body and connecting your body with your mind. Arthritis can be a demanding condition that taxes the body. In times when you are in too much pain to exercise or even walk, the standing pole exercises will help rehabilitate you, help you start feeling better and be a jumping-off point for next-level exercises. At this time, with your specific level of pain tolerance, if you can only do the standing exercises, that is ok. They have been healing people in China for centuries.

Tai Chi

Tai Chi an ancient practice of energy cultivation and body development steeped in traditions of Chinese meditation, breathing exercises and martial arts. Tai Chi is actually a link between QiGong breath-work exercises and kung-fu body training. It is a mind-body discipline that strengthens mind and body while cultivating life force energy, keeping muscles toned, tendons relaxed, the joints supple and blood freely circulating. All of this engenders relaxation, stress relief and pain reduction.

There are eight reasons everyone suffering arthritis should practice Tai Chi:

1. It helps develop balance, preventing falls and fractures common in people suffering arthritis of the hips and knees.

2. It helps build bone density, preventing brittle bones and helping reverse osteoporosis and osteoarthritis.

3. It helps keep muscles toned and fit, preventing flaccidity and weakness while helping support arthritis joints.

4. It helps clear and quiet the mind, reducing stress and anxiety while promoting focus and concentration.

5. It helps regulate the lungs and heart without taxing them, improving wellness and detoxification.

6. It helps burn calories without taxing the joints or stressing the heart, improving fitness levels while aiding in slow and steady weight loss.

7. It helps restore proper range of motion in the wrists, elbows, shoulders, hips, knees and ankles, preventing muscle spasms and neuralgic pain.

8. It helps keep the body active at a sustained rate for a period, moving blood, improving lymph drainage, moving fluids throughout the body and being a source of invigoration.

Many studies have been carried out on the health benefits of practicing Tai Chi, of which there are four main "family" branches: Chen, Yang, Wu, Hao, Sun. All are equally good overall, however, *Wu Style is best suited to those with arthritic hands.*

The Wu style Tai Chi form was developed later specifically for those suffering RA and OA, with symptoms most affecting the fingers and joints of the hands. The hand and wrist postures are modified so they don't stress the arthritis joints of the hands. If the Wu style is not available in your area, you can join any style and reap many useful benefits, just adjust your postures as needed.

Tai Chi also has what are known as "long forms" and "short forms," referring to the number of movements in their sequence. The short form is fine for many people and is easier to learn. However, for those wanting the best of what Tai Chi offers, the long form contains more movements, takes longer and is more interesting overall. I like to think of this art as a "life study" as it combines intellectual activity (learning, remembering and perfecting the sequence), physical activity (the movements and postures themselves), moving meditation (clearing the mind and aligning the body while in motion), and QiGong energy work (combining and coordinating mind, breath and posture in motion).

Because you are holding postures with bent arms and bent knees, Tai Chi is an isometric exercise. However, because you are also moving between postures and connecting them, Tai Chi is also an isotonic exercise. This combination makes Tai Chi able to increase muscle tone and strength while also laying new bone to strengthen bone density, all while improving balance, or "root" as it is known. Thus, Tai Chi is terrific for those with or at risk for osteoporosis and osteopenia, thus reducing chances of falls and broken bones or fractured hips and pelvis.

New studies conducted by Katherine Kerr, a Tai Chi teacher at Harvard Medical School, have found that Tai Chi may also help reduce or prevent disorders of memory and brain function. "Brain plasticity arising from repeated training may be relevant, since we know that brain connections are 'sculpted' by daily experience and practice," says Kerr.

"Tai Chi is a very interesting form of training because it combines a low-intensity aerobic exercise with a complex, learned, motor sequence. Meditation, motor learning and focus have all been shown in numerous studies to be associated with training-related changes – including, in some cases, changes in actual brain structure – in specific cortical regions."

The National Center for Complementary and Alternative Medicine (NCCAM) estimates that nearly three million people in the U.S. practice Tai Chi. What's more, the organization supports the claims that Tai Chi is effective in helping those with "cardiovascular disease, fall prevention, bone health, osteoporosis, osteoarthritis of the knee, rheumatoid arthritis, chronic heart failure, cancer survivors, depression in older people, and symptoms of fibromyalgia." Tai Chi has also been shown to strengthen the immune system.

Yoga

Yoga is an ancient Indian practice of health and well-being that involves holding and moving between various postures, specified breathing methods and achieving altering states of consciousness through meditation. While the broader aim of traditional yogic practices is unifying mind and body with spirit, in the West it has come to be seen as a relaxing or muscle-toning physical activity, depending on yoga style.

One of the basic tenets of chronic pain is that it has both mental and physical origins and manifestations. It is a mind/body phenomenon that requires a mind/body approach. Yoga seems to be a perfect practice to relieve chronic pain. Here's why …

One of the causes of pain is the hypertonicity (tightness) of muscles that constrict blood flow, reduce the amount of fresh oxygen and nutrients in circulation and allow toxins to accumulate in muscle tissue. Yoga is structured around the practice of physical movements that gently move the body. These movements are within the normal ranges of motion and thus do not require great exertion or flexibility, and will not cause sprains and tears while being performed. When the muscles are supple and the blood is moving, pain is reduced and the mental anguish and physical restrictions of that pain are diminished.

Regardless of which yoga method is practiced, studies have confirmed its healing properties. In fact, many studies have found that regular practice of yoga can reduce blood pressure by as much as 15 mm/Hg (millimeters of mercury in blood pressure reading). With extended practice of yoga, a level of fitness is achieved and weight loss experienced, which are also responsible for lowering of blood pressure and reduction of the effects of daily stress. Reduction of stress, lowering of blood pressure, calmness of mind and slowed breathing are all tools that help reduce pain and other symptoms and negative effects of suffering arthritis.

Yoga can be an effective method for decreasing pain by its ability to induce a deep calming effect and slower breathing, which assists in the relaxation of muscles and reduction of trigger points and systemic inflammation. This ancient practice brings down the stress-induced fight or flight response, thereby reducing the levels of the hormones adrenaline and cortisol that are pumping through your system.

Yoga practices, especially those with a spiritual component, also offer practitioners an emotional experience along with their physical movements, fostering feelings of love, kindness, compassion and forgiveness. These feelings alone reduce the way people react to daily stress and the people around them. Stress causes pain, so less stress means less tension in the body and therefore less pain.

The body has learned ways of reacting to stress with protective measures like tension and pain. To overcome those ingrained responses, one needs to retrain the body's response to the mind. Practicing yoga on a weekly or bi-weekly basis has proven effective at doing this. It gives the mind and the body a new pattern of relaxation and quietness. Yoga teaches one to use their mind to observe their body, to control posture, to regulate breathing … all in an effort to allow them to take control of their experiences and how their experiences take hold in the body.

The on-going practice of yoga is transformative. It changes stress and pain responses into healing responses. Over time, it brings one to feel a sense of self-empowerment, vitality and relaxed, stress-free living.

Pain and energy drain comes from tight muscles and tense minds. When the mind is tense, the muscles also become tense. When muscles become tense, they restrict blood flow, decrease range of motion and can cause trigger points. Trigger points are painful dime-sized "knots" deep in the muscle tissue that can cause pain for weeks on end.

Easing mental stresses and physical muscle contractions is a must if you are striving for relief from arthritis. When you are relaxed very little energy is consumed, which allows the body to recharge and repair. These periods of regeneration, just like when sleeping, are vital to proper pain-free functioning.

One natural way of relaxing both mind and body is through regular practice of yoga. By assuming the yoga postures, known as *asanas*, one is able to relax, stretch and tone the body at the same time. How?

Each posture is held for a period of time. This allows toning of the muscles necessary to hold the posture. However, since the postures are all designed to be assumed within the body's normal range of motion, there is little stress or strain. And with low stress, comes slow breathing which relaxes both the mind and the body. Thus, in each moment the yoga *asanas* are held, the person's mind and body relax and recharge. Just like while sleeping, but with the added benefit of gentle, strain-free toning.

When the muscles are toned, they are better able to hold the body in correct posture throughout the day. An imbalance in muscle tone or muscle suppleness is a cause of chronic body pain. If muscle A is strong and muscle B is weak, then A carries the load and B suffers injury while along for the ride. Moreover, neck pain on one side is a sign that the muscles on one side of the neck are either weaker or tenser than the muscles on the other side of the neck. Pain is the result.

So go ahead and take a brisk 20-minute walk and later that day or the next day stand still practicing QiGong for 30 minutes. You may never feel as good as this.

How to Implement These Exercises

It is not necessary to engage in all of these exercises to overcome your arthritis. Choosing even one to begin with is a step in the right direction. Two of them are even better. I recommend beginning with QiGong standing exercises and mindful walking. These can be done at different times of the day without cutting into your daily schedule – you can stand watching the news, waiting in line or talking to friends and you walk everywhere. If you can join a class that offers yoga or Tai Chi, then these can be added to your routine, too. Some people like the solitary time in walking and standing, while others enjoy the group dynamic and support that yoga and Tai Chi classes can offer. Each of them is good and offers similar results, if done correctly. So go ahead and start moving with some safe and low-impact mind-body exercises. They are another of the important pieces in the puzzle of arthritis relief.

Chapter Review

- Make exercise a part of your arthritis relief program, despite the myths to the contrary
- I suggest effective mind/body programs like Walking, QiGong, Tai Chi and Yoga because they are easier to practice in spite of the constant stiffness, inflammation, swelling and pain that accompany arthritis
- Beyond the general health benefits of these exercises, these particular programs help focus your thoughts, emotions, and spirit – reducing stress and anxiety that often comes with arthritis
- Start by choosing one of these programs – it is an important step in the right direction

CHAPTER 14

Bodywork Therapies for Arthritis Relief

Prevention is always the best medicine, but often we do not know something is wrong until its signs and symptoms appear. In the case of arthritis, this is often too late. However, we do have the power to slow the progression of deterioration, and even reverse some of the negative effects, as well as reduce symptoms. Much of the information in the book follows a DIY (do-it-yourself) approach, where you, alone, have the power to activate the remedies. There are times, however, when you will need a little help.

Bodywork therapies are those that utilize the hands of a practitioner on your body to effect change in a positive way. Sometimes the hands-on approach is physical (like with massage) and breaks up connective tissue and relieves trigger points. At other times, the therapy may be interior via injection (such as in prolozone therapy). In each case, you are relying on the healing hands of a trained practitioner to help correct imbalances in your body.

Many who suffer with arthritis find it difficult to exercise because they are either too weak, in too much pain, or have lost too much range of motion. In such cases, attending a series of hands-on bodywork sessions can really help loosen the body, align the system, free the nerves and awaken the energy. In this chapter I'd like to introduce you to some of my favorite hands-on therapies. Read them and decide which one (or two) might work best for you.

Massage Therapy

If done correctly, massage therapy can work wonders for people in pain. It may not always be the best choice, and may not work for everyone, but most people will get great results if the massage therapist has a good understanding of the human body, muscle imbalances and how to work with them.

Massage improves circulation, and this is a big component of pain relief. A clear fluid called lymph circulates around our body's tissues. At the same time, you may have inflammation, which is an immune response to injury or infection that causes pain, redness, heat and swelling in the affected area. People with rheumatoid arthritis (RA) have an incorrect immune response. When lymph and inflammation start to accumulate in the body, the excess fluid puts pressure on blood vessels and circulation decreases, limiting blood flow. As the pressure increases, it irritates the nerves, which cause pain. By helping the body remove excess lymph and inflammation, massage therapy can assist with blood flow, which will reduce the pressure that is irritating the nerves and get rid of your pain.

Massage also provides a number of other benefits, including: relaxing the muscles, improving your range of motion, improving your sleep and increasing your production of endorphins (which will improve your mood). Is it any wonder you feel like a million bucks after a massage?

There are literally hundreds of styles of massage. Which one is best for you will depend on your comfort level. Standard massage is good, moves toxins through the body and is relaxing. But it often does not correct structural problems or offer enough correction in the range of motion, and it is limited range of motion and inflammation that are causing pain.

Trigger Point Therapy

Trigger points are small contraction knots that develop in muscle and tissue when an area of the body is stressed, "frozen," injured or overworked. Sitting for too long or even restricting your movements because of arthritis pain can cause tiny land mines about the size of a dime to erupt deep in your muscle tissue. These are called trigger points, and they can occur in your back, arms, legs and feet.

If you have lingering arthritis pain, or tightness or restriction of certain movements due to arthritis of hips, knee, elbow or hands, it is a good bet that you are experiencing the affects of a trigger point. Massage therapy is usually insufficient when trigger points have a hold on your body and are the cause of your pain. What is needed for relief here is sufficient deep sustained pressure to the "knotted-up area." As the trigger point is worked out, your body will undergo soft tissue release, allowing for increased blood flow, a reduction in muscle spasm, and the break-up of scar tissue. It will also help remove any build-up of toxic metabolic waste.

The good news is, with deep and focused pressure to these areas you can release this pain from your body. However, simply rubbing the surface of the skin with massage oil, a vibrating massager (or using heat) will not heal these pain spots.

What is needed is sufficient deep sustained pressure to the "knotted-up area." As the trigger point is compressed, your body will undergo soft tissue release, allowing for increased blood flow, a reduction in muscle spasm, and the break-up of scar tissue. It also helps remove any build-up of toxic metabolic waste.

Trigger point therapy can be received at the hands of a manual therapist trained in its method. There are also good self-treatment trigger point systems that can work just as well, or better. With a *self-treatment trigger point system*, you can apply pressure to the trigger points every day or several times per day until relief is found.

With trigger point therapy, your body will also undergo a neurological release, reducing the pain signals to the brain and resetting your neuromuscular system to restore its proper function. In other words, everything will again work the way it should.

The basic idea is simply to apply sustained pressure on the trigger point area for a set period of time on a regular basis, usually about 90 seconds per point. A word of caution is needed: if you have RA, do not press directly into the joints or the problem may worsen. Also, trigger point therapy can be painful as the toxins and tissues are released. Be careful and stop if your symptoms worsen.

Thai-Yoga Massage

Thai-yoga massage is a gentle method of hands-on bodywork that is rhythmic and measured. It successfully combines assisted stretching and yoga postures, from either a seated or lying position. In general massage different oils are rubbed on naked body. But because of the nature of the Thai-yoga techniques, the body is fully clothed in loose fitting garments and no oils are used.

The Thai-yoga therapist holds different body parts to gently stretch them, press them or compress them in a slow and rhythmic fashion that releases tension and fosters relaxation. Sometimes, the practitioner (who is usually a petite woman) will hold onto rails and use her feet and body weight to massage the back. The massage follows a sequence from head to toe and releases the energy lines and connective tissue to induce a deep level of somatic correction, relaxation and to free up the body's range of motion.

For those in pain with stiff muscles and joints and with limited range of motion, Thai- yoga massage is a blessing. Unfortunately, its practitioners are few and far between, so be sure to check local massage therapy locations and the Internet.

Tui-Na Therapy

China's 3,000 year tradition of bodywork known as Tui-Na is based on acupuncture theory. It is a rigorous therapy that loosens muscles and joints, relaxes tendons, reduces swelling and relieves pain by promoting the circulation of energy, blood and lymph. It combines techniques of manually pushing, pulling, grasping, pressing and manipulating the muscles, tendons and bones to work through stiffness or injury.

Tui-Na technique apply pressure to the meridians (energy lines) and specific points on them (acu-points), this affects the flow of Qi (vital energy), and helps it move freely and evenly throughout the body. When your body is balanced you feel relaxed and full of energy. You are free from stiffness, aches or pain.

A word of caution, Tui-Na is not for the timid or those in acute pain. It should not to be confused with a nice relaxing massage. It is vigorous and sometimes painful … but then, it is a therapy based on correcting a problem.

Prolozone Therapy

Prolozone therapy is a somewhat recent advance on prolotherapy and is also known as *regeneration injection therapy*. *Prolo* refers to proliferation, or the growth and formation, of new ligament tissue after an irritant has been injected into the damaged ligaments. Ligaments connect bones to bones (tendons connect muscles to bones), and are in essence the shock absorbers of the skeletal system. There is little elastin fiber in ligaments, so when they are weak, injured, damaged or strained they are no longer able to hold the joint structures securely. This causes wearing down of cartilage, rubbing of joint bones, inflammation and pain.

To help correct the structural problem that can cause osteoarthritis and make rheumatoid arthritis and osteoarthritis symptoms worsen, an injection of ozone gas and collagen producing substances is injected into the connective tissue and ligaments around the affected joints. The injection of these substances creates a micro-trauma and controlled inflammation that causes the body to increase circulation, and blood-carrying nutrients and fluids to the damaged area for repair.

While I have not personally undergone prolozone therapy, I have read quite a bit about its successes and am keeping an open mind should I require it in the future. According to Dr. Andrea Purcell, an expert in the therapy, *"Because Prolozone treatments also result in cartilage regeneration, the technique is also remarkably effective even for severe cases of osteoarthritis of the hip or knee. The good thing about Prolozone therapy is that it is not just a treatment for pain. The results can actually represent a permanent fix."*

You can look up more about prolozone therapy on the Internet, and in the Reference section of this book. According to studies, some people require as few as two treatments while more difficult cases require up to seven. If it is as effective at repairing lax joint structures, rebuilding cartilage and stopping pain as it claims to be … give it a try.

How to Choose the Best Method

The above-mentioned alternative therapies are just a handful of those which are able to bring relief from pain and illness by correcting energetic imbalances in the body. They are based on thousands of years of trial-and-error application and have an amazing track record of success.

If you have tried just about everything and are still in pain, then you might want to ditch the mainstream idea of health. Instead, open your mind to these traditional ideas of the body being composed of energy, and that energy vibrating at various frequencies, positively and negatively affecting the mind, body, spirit and organs.

Pain is caused when there is a blockage of this energy. These practices unblock your inherent life energies. Give them a try … pain relief may be just around the corner.

Chapter Review

- Bodywork therapies utilize the hands of a practitioner on your body to effect change in a positive way
- Because of weakness, pain, or lost range of motion, many people don't feel able to exercise, and need a little help moving forward
- Attending a series of bodywork sessions helps to loosen the body, align the system, free the nerves and awaken the energy - giving you the strength to begin
- Of all bodywork therapies, I recommend: Massage, Trigger Point, Thai-Yoga Massage, Tui Na and Prolozone Therapies

CHAPTER 15

Energy Medicine for Arthritis Relief

Everything in the Universe is made up of energy and is vibrating at specific frequencies. There is dense energy, loose energy, erratic energy, calm energy, high frequencies and low frequencies. The human body, too, is nothing if not a physical body constructed of energetic vibrations.

All aspects of health and well-being – especially pain – are tied to energetic frequencies. Problem is, most of us who suffer chronic pain only get the "pain channel" and keep ourselves "tuned in" to it 24/7. Thus the "pain frequency" is maintained and our suffering needlessly prolonged.

If you tune in to an opera channel on your radio, you will get opera, not country music. If you dial your mother on the cell phone, you won't get cousin Betty. If you say bad things about people, you will lose friends. "You reap what you sow," is a good example of the power of attraction, the power of like energy meeting like energy.

If your mental energy is vibrating at a low frequency, you will have trouble studying, thinking or remembering names, places or events. If your physical energy is blocked or sluggish, you will experience aches and pains such as sciatica, headache, fibromyalgia and others. In short:

low frequency = low function and poor health; high frequency = high functioning and good health.

You must change your energetic frequency to feel better and live better.

The Energy Body

Traditional cultures around the world built their healing models on correcting energetic imbalances in the body. The role of Shamans in Siberia, Alaska and Southeast Asia was to eradicate "bad spirits" (i.e., negative energy) from the body to restore physical or mental health in those suffering. The entire pantheon of Chinese and Indian healing practices was built on the premise of energy systems and pathways in the body that, when blocked, cause pain and disease. Clearing these channels or centers of blocked energy (e.g., toxins, spasms), is what restores health to the ill and offers relief to the pain sufferer.

Perhaps the most common term used to talk about human energy is aura. This is a general term used to describe the color, mood or quality of five overlapping energy layers. These layers of energy (or energy bodies) refer to the spiritual, mental, emotional, etheric and physical energies that make up humans.

Energy is developed, stored and moved in the body through the adrenals, the organs, chakra centers and meridian pathways. There is a saying in Traditional Chinese Medicine that tells why we experience pain: "Where there is energy blockage, there is pain. Where energy moves freely, there is no pain."

The key to pain relief and lasting health, then, is to open the energy channels, raise your vibration frequency and keep your energy moving at all times. There are a number of alternative therapies whose primary function is just that.

Polarity Therapy

Like other energy medicine methodologies, polarity therapy sees the human body as comprising "life energy." However, polarity therapy takes the view that the energy body is in a state of constant "pulsation," with positive and negative poles and a neutral position. These poles and position form a kind of energetic "template" along the body, on which a practitioner can apply touch and pressure to alter the pulsations and derive pain relief and better general states of health.

While it shares common ideas with acupressure and QiGong, polarity therapy is more aligned with Indian Ayurvedic medicine and modern osteopathic and chiropractic theories of the body. When people have gone through the complete series of acupuncture or QiGong treatments recommended by their practitioner, and have not found substantial relief, polarity therapy may be the next best modality to embrace. Oftentimes, a person's polarity (positive/negative energy poles) is reversed, and one or more polarity sessions can correct this.

Quantum Touch®

The new kid on the block, in terms of hands-on energy work, is called Quantum Touch®. It is both a method for individuals to work on themselves and for practitioners to work on those in need of its healing potential. It does this through simple methods whereby life force energy is amplified and entrained. This process helps the body facilitate its own healing process.

The claims Quantum Touch® to relieve chronic pain was put to the test through an eight-week pilot study in which the investigators used 12 volunteer adult patients (men and women ages 18 to 64) who were randomly selected and randomly assigned to an experimental and control group of six volunteers in each group. Both groups were blindfolded and received hands-on touch; however, only the experimental group was given the Quantum Touch® energy. What was made very clear through the research was that Quantum Touch® healing is effective and has a positive impact on clients in the area of chronic musculoskeletal pain. This holistic modality, like others before it, can now offer itself to the world of health and wellness as a viable method of pain management with documented evidence of its impact and effectiveness.

Reiki

Reiki is a Japanese energy technique for reducing stress and inducing relaxation to help promote the free-flow of energy in the body. Reiki is both a non-touch and a "laying on of hands" by a practitioner for its benefits to be gained.

Reiki practitioners lay their hands on patients in various configurations that are modeled on ancient Tibetan and Chinese powerful healing symbols. It is believed that re-creating these symbols on the body will allow

"God's energy" to flow from the Universe, through the practitioner and into the patient. This energy, which is vibrating at a high frequency, will lift the low energy of the sufferer to relieve pain and illness.

Reiki has become a popular healing modality among nurses in hospitals. The patient does not have to be awake for them to administer a few minutes of healing touch. It may be the easiest of the energy healing systems to find a practitioner and also feels really good. However, of all the methods I have personally studied and been treated with, Reiki seems to have the least corrective benefits. Good for relaxation and acute symptomatic relief, but not as effective for long-term relief based on being a truly corrective body therapy.

Jin Shin Jyutsu

Similar to its Chinese cousins, jin shin jyutsu aims to balance the physical and mental energies in the body. It views the body as being composed of a trinity of energy pathways that, when functioning properly, harmonize mind, body and spirit.

Jin shin jyutsu's healing ability is based on manipulating and opening 26 energy points, known as the "safety energy factors." When activated through finger pressure, these points unblock stagnant energy, relieve tension and allow energy to flow freely in the body. Like acupressure, patients can both receive treatment from a practitioner, or they can learn self-pressure methods to regulate their own energy centers.

QiGong Therapy

QiGong refers to specific health exercises or techniques for regulating the body, mind and breath. They involve visualization, movement, posture and self-massage to effect interior balance and thus positive changes in health.

Regular practice of QiGong aids in regulating the functions of the central nervous system. Along with exercising and controlling one's mind and body, QiGong influences one's physical states and pathological conditions. Concurrently, the practice of QiGong emits latent energy within the human body, enabling the practitioner to use them to their fullest potential. Regular practice increases the body's ability to adapt to and defend against the natural/physical environment in which we live.

The primary use of QiGong today is to improve one's health, thus extending life. This is known as medical or healing QiGong, of which there are three subdivisions:

1) Applied clinical therapy, whereby a Chinese doctor emits (projects) his own qi into a patient's body to effect a cure;

2) Self-regulating exercises, whereby a person chooses a QiGong program and practices the exercises over a period of at least 100 days to improve his or her own health;

3) A combination of clinical QiGong treatments from a doctor and an individual's personal self-regulating QiGong training program. Within the self-practice method, exercises are done in any

combination of three ways: static postures, slow movements, meditation and breathing exercises.

Acupuncture

Acupuncture is no longer the backroom healing art of Chinatown immigrants. On the contrary, not only is it a household word, but it is extremely popular among women in their 40s and 50s and sports competitors. Moreover, mainstream medical doctors are increasingly offering acupuncture in their offices as an adjunct to their own practices.

But many people are still leery of this 5,000-year-old tradition. They wonder if it is real or just new age hype. The World Health Organizations (WHO) has vetted this ancient Chinese healing tradition and announced that acupuncture is suitable for treating the following conditions:

- **Ear, Nose and Throat Disorders:** toothaches, pain after tooth extraction, gingivitis, acute or chronic otitis, acute sinusitis, acute rhinitis, nasal catarrh and acute tonsillitis.
- **Respiratory Disorders:** asthma, bronchitis, colds and allergies.
- **Gastrointestinal Disorders:** esophageal and cardio spasm, hiccup, gastroptosis, acute or chronic gastritis, sour stomach, chronic duodenal ulcers, acute or chronic colonitis, acute bacillary dysentery, constipation, diarrhea and paralytic ileus.

- **Eye Disorders:** acute conjunctivitis, central retinitis, nearsightedness (in children) and cataracts.

- **Neurological and Muscular Disorders:** headaches, migraines, trigeminal neuralgia, facial paralysis (within the first three to six months), post-stroke paresis, peripheral neuritis, neurological bladder dysfunction, bed wetting, intercostal neuralgia, cervical syndrome, frozen shoulder, tennis elbow, sciatica, low back pain and osteoarthritis.

In other words, acupuncture is effective for not only arthritis, but many of the pain disorders associated with it.

Acupressure is the non-invasive and non-needle offspring of acupuncture, the therapy where thin needles are inserted into the skin to correct energetic imbalances. Both work on the same theory, and in both cases, the practitioner will either "needle" or apply finger pressure to specific points (acu points) on the body. Using a correct "prescription" of points, the practitioner can in effect change the energy in a patient, open their channels and help their energy move more freely.

Acupuncture and acupressure are both widely practiced today and worth looking into. They have been around for 5,000 years and have helped millions of people. The acupuncture needles work like antennae puling bioelectric energy from the atmosphere into the body to correct energy imbalances within the body's meridian channels.

Frequency Specific Microcurrent FSM Therapy

Frequency-specific microcurrent (FSM) therapy specifically treats myofacial neuropathic pain reducing inflammatory cytokines (polypeptide regulators). In other words, it helps reduce trigger points and fascial constrictions that cause pain, sensations like "pins and needles," coldness or burning, numbness or itching caused by a damaged or diseased sensory system, as is common in arthritis.

FSM is a non-invasive therapy that requires the use of a two-channel microamperage current device, which can be purchased online. The treatment requires two separate channels of voltage (13Hz and 396Hz) to be connected to the patient while attempting to move their affected limbs to their utmost range of motion. Clinical studies show that these specific frequencies, when used simultaneously, can effectively treat nerve and muscle pain, reduce inflammation and clear scar tissue. Other frequencies help reduce the pain associated with kidney stones, and aid in healing of asthma, liver dysfunction, irritable bowel syndrome (IBS) and other conditions.

Pulsed Electromagnetic Frequency PEMF Therapy

For many, the idea such a thing as harmful electromagnetic frequency (EMF) smog has never crossed their minds. If you cannot see it, it does not exist, right?

Wrong. This smog is all around us, every day, everywhere we go. It originates from the frequencies of cell towers, Wi-Fi in cafes, cell and cordless phones, High Definition televisions, laptop computers, microwaves and especially in our vehicles. EMFs are making us ill and killing us slowly by breaking down the very structure of our cells. There is no escaping it.

Martin Blank, Ph.D. of Columbia University says, "Cells in the body react to low level EMFs and produce a biochemical stress response. Our safety standards are inadequate. People need to sit up and pay attention."

We are immersed in a sea of EMF radiation. It comes from cordless phones and base stations, cell phones and towers, electrical appliances, computers, fluorescent lighting, Bluetooth devices, Wi-Fi installations and more than 2,000 satellites for GPS and TV and radio communications.

"New research is suggesting that nearly all of the human plagues which emerged in the 20th century, including leukemia in children, female breast cancer, malignant melanomas, immune system disorders, asthma and others, can be tied in some way to our use of electricity."

Here's a breakdown of the negative health effects of prolonged EMF exposure. That is, exposure over a scant two milligauss:

- Interferes with our body's intracellular communications and cell membrane function.

- Reduces hemoglobin surface area and interferes with blood's ability to carry oxygen and nutrients into our cells and take the waste products out.
- Activates proto-oncogenes (which can cause cancer).
- Increases permeability of the blood-brain barrier and affects intra-cerebral pressure, which some believe seems to bring on Alzheimer's, Parkinson's, autism, multiple sclerosis and other neurodegenerative disorders.
- Causes DNA breaks and chromosome aberrations.
- Increases free radical production.
- Causes cell stress and premature aging.
- Causes changes in brain function, including memory loss, learning impairment, headaches and fatigue.
- Reduces melatonin secretion. Melatonin is responsible for sleep patterns and helps protect the body against cancer, among other things.
- Causes many microorganisms living in the human body to generate increased levels of their own toxins, affecting people's health in myriad ways.

In a nutshell, each of our cells is surrounded by something called a phospholipid bi-layer membrane, commonly known as the cell membrane. Embedded in the cell membrane are numerous proteins that act as receptors for various molecules, including enzymes. These receptors translate the positive/negative signals on the cell's exterior into its interior, and these signals then trigger various biological processes.

When we're affected by external electromagnetic fields, the high-speed positive/negative polarity switching within these fields, from hundreds to millions of times per second, interferes with our cells' internal signaling process. Basically, it confuses them and they become paralyzed.

A product recently permitted into the United States claims it can reverse this damage this in only eight minutes, two to three times a day. It's called the MRS2000, and is a German-engineered medical device that uses pulsed, healthy EMFs to counter the debilitating effects of today's EMF smog and help bring people to optimal health.

It turns out (much like the discovery of both good and bad cholesterol), that certain EMFs are actually good for us. In fact, we can't live without them. As a result, much research has gone into refining pulsed EMF therapy and the results are impressive.

Paul Rosch, M.D., of New York Medical College, went on record to say, "While EMFs are responsible for quite a bit of damage, don't throw the baby out with the bathwater. Pulsed electromagnetic frequency (PEMF) therapies have been shown to be beneficial for stress related disorders, for anxiety, insomnia, arthritis, depression and more. They also may be safer and more effective than drugs."

Thousands of clinical studies are proving its value, and PEMF therapy is beginning to get the recognition it deserves. While experts may not all agree on what EMF exposure levels cause what health issues, the dearth of evidence out there suggests we would be foolish not to apply the precautionary principle and reduce our exposure. Using the MRS2000 could be a big step in the right direction.

Chapter Review

- The entire Universe, including the human body, is made of energy, vibrating at specific frequencies.
- All aspects of health and well-being – including pain – are tied to energetic frequencies
- Unfortunately, those in chronic pain are "tuned in" to the "pain channel," keeping themselves focused solely on their pain
- You can and must change your energetic frequency to feel better and live better
- You can shift your energy with practices and methods like: Polarity Therapy, Quantum Touch, Reiki, Jin Shin Jyutsu, QiGong Therapy, Acupuncture, FSM Therapy, and PEMF Therapy

CHAPTER 16

Stress Reduction, Relaxation and Sleep for Arthritis Relief

Stress is one of the leading causes of illness in the United States. Nearly 66 percent of all signs and symptoms presented in doctors' offices in the U.S. are stress induced. Most people who suffer arthritis also suffer the ill effects of stress. The inability to do what they used to be able to do, coupled with pain and inflammation, creates physical, psychological and emotional stress.

The Nasty Effects of Stress

The effects of stress include nail biting, anxiety, a racing mind, obsessive thoughts, compulsive behavior, unending worry, muscle tension and spasm, poor appetite or too great an appetite, digestive disorders, constipation, insomnia, poor blood flow, belabored breathing, neck pain, shoulder tension and the possible onset or continuation of bad habits such as dependence on alcohol, drugs, painkillers, food and caffeine.

Any one of these things by itself can trigger any number of different types of illnesses. But when these forces of antagonism are combined (as they generally are when triggered by stress), the health problems often become chronic and insufferable. In short, stress makes arthritis worse and arthritis causes more stress. It is a vicious cycle that needs to be broken. Before I show you how, let's look at the psychology of stress to better understand the solutions I offer.

The Psychology of Stress

Stress is an interesting phenomenon. It means different things to different people. What we each individually consider to be stressful is largely a matter of our perception. Our perceptions are our realities and so what we think is posing a threat is actually doing so by virtue of our established belief system. Moreover, there are many kinds of stressors – physical (the response to being frightened), emotional (loss of a loved one), psychological (obsessive thoughts), spiritual (loss of faith) and psychosomatic (the need for attention).

Physiologically, stress is responsible for initiating the fight-or-flight response in the face of perceived danger. This means that when we are confronted with a danger, our body automatically prepares us to deal with the coming stressful situation by focusing our attention, pumping more blood into our muscles and sending adrenaline through our system to ready it for action. It is precisely this response that helps protect the body and return it again to homeostasis. However, too much stress, or stress left unresolved for too long a time, can lead to biological damage.

You see, at the onset of perceived danger the body is quickly jolted into fight-or-flight mode, which means stress hormones such as adrenaline and cortisol are pumped into the bloodstream. However, at the conclusion of the danger episode, the body does not automatically calm down and return to homeostasis. In fact, it takes a great deal of time for the body to return to so-called normal conditions. But often this cannot happen because another stressor may present itself (e.g., sitting in traffic, standing in line at the bank, missing a deadline) and this sends our body into "code red" mode all over again.

The effects of such prolonged or recurring stress is that it keeps the autonomic nervous system from balancing, which can lead to problems with the gastrointestinal tract, the digestive system, the respiratory system and the neuroendocrine system. It breaks down the body's immune system, which needs to be strong and stable for those suffering rheumatoid arthritis (RA). Stress can also lead to depression, anxiety, muscle tension, insomnia and body pain. All of these are known triggers of various mental and physical (mind/body) illnesses and diseases, including arthritis.

The Arthritis Relief Action Plan offers many solutions for each aspect of the puzzle. In terms of stress reduction the plan includes a mind-body approach for long-term success. In the short term, there are simpler solutions to bust the stress as it arises. Here are 10 possible solutions.

10 Simple Stress Busters

The idea behind living stress-free is to remove the things in your life that cause you to be stressed. Of course, this is easier said than done, but it is truly the only way to not have stress. Here are 10 simple things you can do daily to reduce the symptoms of stress.

1. Walk outside for at least 20 continuous minutes every day
2. Quiet the mind and calm the nerves with meditation
3. Take 10 deep belly breaths every hour
4. Drink plenty of pure water – at least 10 glasses a day
5. Avoid sugar and caffeine in all forms
6. Regulate sleep and wake cycles to a consistent daily routine
7. Prioritize your life, work, family and personal time and activities
8. Do six shoulder shrugs whenever you are tense
9. Realize that when people criticize and judge they are labeling an "image" of you and not you personally
10. Realize that you are worth so much more than the sum of your titles, money and belongings

A good stress-relief program should be followed when controlling for arthritis. Good programs generally include various forms of meditation, diet, exercise, QiGong, yoga, bodywork and sleeping. Each of these is actually a component of our overall arthritis relief program. Stress is a monster that really takes its toll. Let's look at how relaxation and meditation can reduce your stress and also change your genes.

Changing States of Consciousness

Often, when folks think of practices like meditation, or yoga and Tai Chi (discussed in Chapter 15), they often think of esoteric practices of past masters and sages. When psychologists began researching these practices, they noticed how the mind (or mental state) of the practitioner was able to affect the body (or physical state). These mind states were often referred to as "altered states." In addition to deep relaxation, they produced excited visions, mental clarity, apparent insanity and states in which physical pains were not felt. Hmm … intriguing.

Internal and external deep relaxation of the body is one healthful side effect of these practices. For some reason all the various "altered states" and "energy" practices produce an underlying state of relaxation. This occurs in different techniques that may originate in widely diverse belief or religious systems.

This "relaxation response" was discovered across all methodologies by Dr. Herbert Benson decades ago. His research using the scientific method proves its value on a cellular level.

The Relaxation Response

Herbert Benson, MD, is a pioneer researcher who has studied mind-body methods and medicine from the perspective of a Western scientific model. He spent time in China researching the effects of QiGong. More than 20 years ago, he participated in conversations between scientists and Buddhists initiated by the 14th Dalai

Lama. These discussions were organized by the Mind & Life Institute.

According to Benson, the relaxation response is "a physical state of deep rest that changes the physical and emotional responses to stress … and the opposite of the fight-or-flight response." The fight-or-flight response, an elevated state of excitation that causes harm in the body when it goes on too long, can be reduced or countered by meditation.

Benson proved that practicing meditative techniques to induce the relaxation response creates a healthier environment within the body. Heart rate, breath rate, blood pressure and body pain are all reduced through this type of relaxation. But Benson also investigated to see if the meditative state of deep relaxation had prolonged effects on human biology that were not merely temporary. This has intriguing implications for autoimmune diseases like rheumatoid arthritis.

The Scientific Proof

In his book "Relaxation Revolution," Benson describes his research into the significant biological differences between meditators and the rest of the population. In other words, he set out to prove or disprove scientifically the effects of the relaxation response on the genetic structure within the body.

He devised a study that looked at two groups of 19 individuals. The first group consisted of people not involved in any form of mind-body practice. The second group encompassed individuals who had been involved in mind-body practices (like meditation, yoga and repetitive prayer) for an average of 9.4 years.

In the study, Benson and colleagues used highly sophisticated gene-analyzing technology to microanalyze the activity of all 54,000 genes within both groups of participants. Blood was drawn from each person, and samples were placed in a centrifuge to separate its components. The scientists then harvested the red and white blood cells containing the genetic material (genes, DNA, RNA). Eventually, they were able to isolate all 54,000 genes and identify which were actively expressed.

Dramatic Differences

Benson found "dramatic differences" between the group of experienced mind-body practitioners and the other group. "Specifically, 2,209 genes in the experienced practitioners were being expressed differently than the same genes in the inexperienced participants. The probability of this result being due to chance was less than five in 100."

These results gave the world scientific proof that ancient practices like yoga, meditation, Tai Chi, QiGong, religious chanting and others were not just games and pastimes but real contributors to the health and mental states of those participating in them. He proved scientifically what others knew intuitively and felt experientially: that these practices aren't based in random beliefs or wishful thinking, but have profound effects on our genetic structure.

Benson and colleagues found that the specific genes that acted differently within those who practice meditation or some form of mind-body method "have been associated with stress-related medical problems, including unhealthful regulation of immune responses; various forms of inflammation, premature aging, including thinning of the cortex of the brain; and other health conditions that may involve oxidative stress." These health issues can be reduced or reversed through meditation, yoga, prayer and other methods both religious and secular that aim to trigger the relaxation response. This response can provide a significant net gain in reversing and preventing further damage caused by arthritis, and in the reduction of its symptoms.

Benson's Simple Meditation

From his research into and analysis of a plethora of mind-body practices around the world, Benson distilled their essence into a simple, secular method for bringing the practitioner into a deep state of physiological relaxation. His method is clear and easy to do, and it is concerned only with the relaxation response (not spiritual enlightenment or other goals).

Benson's method contains two parts:

Part 1

For 10 to 20 minutes, continuously repeat a word, phrase, sound, prayer or movement and align it with your natural breathing cycle.

Part 2

When outside noises or thoughts intrude during

practice, simply take notice of them and avoid judgment or response to them. Simply return to the task at hand.

These two parts are the basic guidelines. There are nine steps to the actual practice that helps create a deep state of relaxation when the relaxation response can be induced. The steps of Benson's relaxation response are:

1. Choose the focus of your meditation (a single word, prayer, movement, etc.).
2. Lie down or sit still in a comfortable position.
3. Close your eyes.
4. Relax your muscles. (This can be done progressively, scanning from the toes to the tip of the head.)
5. Focus on your breathing. (Observe your breath as it moves in and out of your body, without stressing over it.)
6. Silently repeat the chosen word or prayer or do the selected motion with each exhalation.
7. Repeat this process of focusing on your breath while repeating the word or movement for 10 to 20 minutes.
8. After completion, sit quietly for a few moments, eyes closed, to reawaken into the world.
9. Do not stress or overthink how well you are meditating or are able to hold the phrase or observe the breath. Just allow it to happen.

Gradual Progress

Like anything else, progress is made slowly and gradually over time. It is advised to practice this meditative exercise twice per day, in the early morning and late evening before bed. In this way you relax at night for optimal repair and wake refreshed and ready to start the day in the best state possible. Continue the daily practice for an extended period of time (months and even years), and the results you experience may be life changing.

While many like to meditate first thing in the morning to begin the day in a level place, I like to meditate before going to sleep. This way I have uninterrupted time and have nothing pressing to keep my mind alert for after the session. And once the relaxation response is activated, I allow myself to drift off into a deep and restful sleep, where healing occurs.

Whether you do it in the morning or evening, getting restful sleep is essential to physical repair and stress reduction. In fact, when you sleep your body metabolizes the harmful stress hormones that cause pain and weight gain. So let us now look at how improper sleeping can cause you additional pain and how correct sleeping can improve your quality of life and help you overcome arthritis.

Restful Sleep Reduces Pain and Inflammation

As a person who has suffered from excruciating headaches and body pain for the better part of 30 years, let me assure you that sound sleep is a wonder pill nobody should do without. Not only is sleep a fundamental human need, it is a necessity that no one who experiences aches or pains of any kind should ever take for granted.

Sleep is so important, in fact, we naturally fall asleep when our body tells our brain that certain essential chemicals have been depleted and our muscles and ligaments are tired and in need of restoration.

The growing problem is that many of us rely on legal stimulants such as coffee, tea and sodas to force ourselves to continue plugging away. Work, after all, cannot be held back by pleading and there are just not enough hours in the week. The result?

We stay up too late, get up too early, and to do this we consume unhealthy amounts of toxic substances – night after night after night.

The net problem is that for the better part of our adult lives, many people are both sick AND tired and this is constantly taking its toll. Let's look at some of the damage caused simply by not going to sleep when we are tired.

Lack of sleep causes: poor concentration, slower reaction times, decreased performance levels, less ability to learn and compartmentalize new skills and knowledge, more frequent memory lapses, increases in simple injuries and accidents, adverse changes in moods and behaviors, increased frequency of headaches, neck and shoulder pain, backaches, fatigue and overload of toxic consumption.

This happens because during restful sleep our body is actually working to repair itself. The liver purifies blood, the muscles repair, serotonin increases. Without ample sleep, these things do not happen at optimal levels.

In our natural circadian rhythm, or biological clock, sleep is set to take over during the evening hours. We are genetically programmed to get up and lie down with the sun. It was the invention of artificial sources of light (candles and bulbs) that began our stressed-out drive for more working hours at the expense of much-needed rest.

What's the big deal, you ask, if you sleep only a few hours per night? You can always drink coffee, take caffeine pills, cat naps … life is good. Well, not really. Did you know that in clinical tests rats die within a few weeks of sleep deprivation?

Chronic fatigue, adrenal fatigue, attention deficit disorder, chronic migraine and headache, body aches and pain, mental illness, depression and anxiety are all in part caused – or made worse – by lack of sleep. And lack of sleep causes lower levels of the neurotransmitter serotonin, placing you at risk for depression and suicidal thoughts. And these are not far behind in those who suffer arthritis.

Here are some simple tips for overcoming insomnia:

- Do not consume ANY sugar or caffeine after 6 p.m.
- Stop working at least two hours before bedtime.
- Turn off the computer and television at least one hour before bedtime.

- Make sure your sleeping quarters are as dark and silent as possible. Studies have shown that those in darker and quieter spaces tend to sleep through the night more deeply than others .
- Establish a sleep/wake schedule, and stick to it.
- Make a bedtime routine. Change into pajamas, brush your teeth, set out clothes for the morning, even jot down any last thoughts but promise yourself to revisit them tomorrow, then turn off the light … breathe deeply, relax, sleep tight.
- If a racing mind is nagging, slow your breath and focus on the sensation of air as it passes through your nose. This will derail those busy thoughts to help you drift off.

For those who exercise at night, flip the schedule. It's keeping you up by moving blood and energy through your system. Researcher at Stanford University School of Medicine found that adults ages 55 to 75 who engaged in 20 to 30 minutes of low-impact exercise (like walking) every other day in the afternoon fell asleep in half their normal time. What's more, their sleep duration increased on average by one full hour.

What does all this mean? Your mom was right. Good health begins as easily and naturally as going out for a walk and putting in plenty of sack time. Try, if possible, for a straight eight hours. And maybe think about buying a new set of sheets, to celebrate the new healthier, happier sounder-sleeping you.

Wrong Sleeping Causes Pain

The power of restorative rest and sleep is strong and wide reaching. In fact, symptoms of diseases like arthritis, fibromyalgia, migraine headaches, chronic fatigue and the flu are decreased while we sleep. But did you know that improper sleep can be a cause of pain and suffering? Poor sleeping posture is the reason for this.

While there are many ways to sleep and many products that allow us to sleep in those ways, there are actually only two healthy positions for engaging in sound slumber. Before we look at those let's review some of the more common sleeping positions and why they are harmful to the body.

Stomach Sleeping – Stomach sleepers, well, sleep on their stomachs. Usually they have one or both arms extended over their heads, their face turned either to the left or right side and one leg is generally bent.

There are so many problems with this posture. First, sleeping with the arms extended over the head raises the shoulders into the neck, causing cramping, poor circulation and pain. It also skews the trapezius muscles and skeletal system, compressing the thoracic outlet where the brachial plexus of nerves from the neck travel down the arms to the hands.

Second, when the arms are raised the nerves are irritated and nerve function is either inhibited or excited. It's a neurological and vascular response that affects the brachial plexus of nerves that travels from the neck and down the arms. The effect is tingling and/or numbness in the arms or hands. Ever wake up with pins and needles in the hands or a "dead" arm? This may be why.

Third, sleeping with the neck turned to one side creates unbalanced muscles, wherein one side is hypertonic (contracted) and the other is hypotonic (extended). This leads to neck strain, cramping, pain and often headaches.

Fourth, the bent leg stretches one leg and hip all night, while the other remains prone. Again, we have imbalance that can lead to hip pain and leg pain.

And fifth, stomach sleeping offers too little support for the abdomen, allowing the stomach to fall forward and the lumbar region of the back to sag. This can make your gut seem bigger than it is, simply because of poor sleeping posture. It also created spinal compression and lower back pain. By extension, there can be spinal nerve irritation that radiates through your arthritis hip or knees, this increasing pain and/or reducing the healing response.

Comfortable or not, this position has to go.

Back Sleeping – Back sleepers are on to something. The back is one of the two best ways to sleep because it can offer solid support for your entire musculoskeletal system.

Problems arise for back sleepers, however, when they do not place pillows under their knees. If you are lying on your back and your legs are straight, there is insufficient support for the lower back allowing it to arch too high.

If you sleep on your back with one leg bent, you probably experience the same hip, lower back and/or knee strain and pain as do the stomach sleepers who sleep in this way.

You should always place two pillows under your knees for support and one pillow under your head. Keep in mind, too, that pillows are for sleeping support, and not just for comfort. Your head should be placed squarely on your pillow, and the pillow should be pulled down enough so that it touches your shoulders. If your pillow is not touching your shoulders you run the risk of not supporting the cervical vertebrae and neck muscles and pain can result from spasm or nerve impingement.

Side Sleeping – Side sleeping gets my vote for best sleeping position, if done correctly. To begin, side posture should mimic the fetal position. That is, both knees bent and with hands held close to the body. This is a normal and inherent sleeping posture.

Errors in side sleeping occur when one leg overlaps the other. This causes an imbalance in the hips that can lead to tightness and pain in the hip flexors, IT band, low back and knees.

Another common error is sleeping with hands under or over the head and scrunching the pillow so your head is elevated. Symptoms from this can include neck and shoulder pain, stiffness, headaches, tingly or numbness in the arms or hands.

Side sleeping is the best because it allows the body to maintain a proper and corrective posture for several hours. What you should do is place a pillow between your knees to create proper distance between them, thus keeping the hips in proper balance. The legs must be parallel, so the hips remain square and there is no strain on the low back. A pillow should be placed under the head and pulled to the shoulder for optimal neck support. The hands should be parallel and below the eyes.

The caveat here is that if you have an arthritic hip, sleeping on that side will aggravate the condition because your body weight is on it. If you have one arthritic hip, it is easy to just side sleep with the other side down. If both hips are arthritic, then sleep on your back with pillows under your knees.

Who knew there was so much to sleeping posture? Try these corrections, then after a while your daily neck strain, shoulder pain, headaches, hip and low back pain and arm tingling may just start to correct itself. In addition, please read the next section on how restful sleep reduces pain and inflammation.

Chapter Review

- Stress is one of the leading causes of illness in the United States, and accounts for almost 66 percent of doctors' office visits
- The effects of stress are numerous, and while a natural response, an excess of stress will lead to biological damage
- Prolonged or recurring stress keeps the autonomic nervous system from balancing, which can lead to problems with the gastrointestinal tract, the digestive system, the respiratory system and the neuroendocrine system. It breaks down the body's immune system, which needs to be strong and stable for those suffering rheumatoid arthritis (RA).
- Stress can also lead to depression, anxiety, muscle tension, insomnia and body pain. All of these are known triggers of various mental and physical (mind/body) illnesses and diseases, including arthritis.
- Review the 10 Simple Stress Busters in this chapter again and often
- You can derail the negative effects of stress by changing your state of consciousness to induce deep mental and physical relaxation
- Never underestimate the power of restful sleep as a way to reduce pain and inflammation, all while allowing your body to repair itself
- Actively practice the Seven Simple Tips for overcoming insomnia on page 194

CHAPTER 17

Resolving Negative Thoughts and Emotions for Arthritis Relief

For some people, the cause of acute and chronic pain is not related to a traumatic injury or arthritis. For these people, no matter what they try and no matter what type of practitioner they see for their pain, they still suffer. The problem could very well be psychosomatic, meaning *the issue is related to both mind and body and how they interact.*

What I am talking about is how negative thought patterns can keep you from recovering and make your condition worse — by amplifying the pain and other symptoms. They do this by creating a mild oxygen deprivation in the body that hampers the health of cells and muscles. This causes restriction of blood vessels and contraction of muscles. You know, it's those tight shoulders you feel when your boss reprimands you or your loved one yells and you hold back negative feelings. It's the repression of such negative feelings that does the damage, or at least initiates a sequence of things that later causes damage (like overeating and weight gain, lack of exercise and stiff muscles, etc.).

If the physical body has been treated in every safe way imaginable but to no avail, perhaps looking at your thoughts and your emotions – a psychosomatic cause – may be the next logical step for you. Below we look at three of the safest, easiest and most power mind/body systems for eradicating chronic pain and associated with negative thoughts and emotions.

The Sedona Method

Pioneered by Lester Levenson, the Sedona Method is a powerful yet easy-to-learn technique that teaches you how to "let go" of unwanted emotions in an instant. These emotions cause ill health, pain and suffering. In essence, The Sedona Method consists of a series of questions you ask yourself that lead your awareness to what you are feeling in the moment and gently guide you into the experience of "letting go."

This method is easy to do because there are only a few steps necessary to accomplish the release of new or decades-old pent-up negative emotions. With so many successes, this again points to the vital role that the mind and emotions play in the pain cycle and ill effects we suffer in our bodies – those psychosomatic illnesses.

The effectiveness of The Sedona Method has been validated by respected scientific researchers at major universities and the MONY Corporation. In fact, if you're not feeling happy, confident and relaxed at least 90 percent of the time, chances are your ailments are manifestations of these less-than-great emotions.

Sedona literature puts it this way: "It is our limiting emotions that prevent us from creating and maintaining the lives that we choose. We abdicate our decision-making ability to them. We even imagine that our emotions can dictate to us who we are supposed to be. This is made apparent in our use of language. Have you ever said to someone, 'I am angry,' or, 'I am sad'? When we speak like this, we are saying to those around us and to ourselves, without realizing it, that we are our anger, or we are our grief. We relate to others and ourselves as though we are our feelings. In fact, we even invent whole stories of why we feel the way we feel in order to justify or explain this misperception of our identity."

If you've tried other mental techniques, therapy or meditation, you know it is difficult to create change. But The Sedona Method's "releasing method" operates on the "feeling" level, which makes it easy to do. It teaches you to "let go" of years of mental programs and accumulated feelings in just seconds.

Emotional Freedom Technique (EFT)

Based on a method known as Thought Field Therapy and also on acupuncture theory, EFT relieves pain and illness by addressing the connection between your body's subtle energies, your emotions and your health.

This therapeutic method is similar to transcranial magnetic stimulation but goes deeper in its explanation of what causes the emotional imbalances. EFT practitioners believe that disturbances in your energy field cause the negative emotions, which then cause your symptoms. Essentially, EFT teaches methods of looking in specific directions, touching and pressing your face and arms in certain places to open the energy channels and rebalance what is out of balance. This then allows your body to return to normal functioning and for your signs and symptoms to decrease or disappear.

It appears that anyone can learn and use Emotional Freedom Technique by taking a course, reading a book or going through the tutorials on EFT websites.

Keep in mind that the role of the mind and the emotions is central to perpetuating and holding that pain in the body. If you have not tried them before or have tried and failed at them, please take a fresh look at the healing methods based on psychosomatic causes of pain and illness. You just may find the release and relief you have been looking for.

But no matter which methods or natural remedies you pursue, remember that health and well-being are rooted in positive, healthy lifestyle choices.

Tension Myositis Syndrome (TMS)

Tension Myositis Syndrome (TMS) is a relatively unknown and somewhat recent health diagnostic category. It was first theorized in the 1970s by John Sarno, M.D., as being a psychosomatic or mind-body disorder: a musculoskeletal neurological disorder created by the mind and emotions that changes one's physiology and causes pain and other symptoms.

Essentially, it is believed that stress and repressed emotions like anger and anxiety are the root cause of chronic back pain and a host of other disorders (discussed below). The theory of TMS, though not widely accepted in mainstream medicine yet, contends that repressed emotional triggers affect the nervous system which, in turn, slows blood flow to muscles, nerves and connective tissue. It basically causes a reaction or process that starves the body of oxygen, causing pain. This pain then becomes the location of focus and concern, alleviating the need (superficially) for dealing with the stress, anxiety and other emotional issues at hand. TMS case studies show that as the emotional components are dealt with successfully, the physical ailments that were heretofore intractable disappear almost instantly.

While pain in general (low back pain in particular) seems to be the most common symptom of TMS, it is not the only one. Generalized stiffness and numbness and tingling in the body or limbs are also associated with the syndrome. Flare-ups from painful to severe come and go at different times, showing the correlation of symptoms to (perhaps) the emotional upset state of the individual at any given time.

Many who experience the problems of chronic pain, tension headache, fibromyalgia, irritable bowel syndrome (IBS), constipation, arm pain, temporal mandibular joint dysfunction (TMJD) and tinnitus (ringing in the ears) have had difficulty finding relief or cure from mainstream approaches. They may have the basis or root of their symptoms in TMS.

As a mind-body practitioner myself and as someone who has suffered debilitating headaches and musculoskeletal pain for most of my life, I have always thought the psychosomatic (mind-body) connection plays a central role in our daily state of health. What I find intriguing about TMS is its theory of equivalence; it offers a connection not generally made in the mainstream or alternative health communities. Here are four short passages from Sarno's book "Healing Back Pain" that are interesting, informative and thought-provoking:

- "TMS is equivalent to peptic ulcer, spastic colitis, constipation, tension headache, migraine headache cardiac palpitations, eczema, allergic rhinitis (hay fever), prostatitis (often), ringing in the ears (often), and dizziness (often)."

- "I believe these disorders are interchangeable and equivalent of each other because many of them are found to occur historically in patients with TMS, sometimes at the same time, but often in tandem."

- "Equivalence is also suggested by the fact that patients often report resolution of one of these disorders when the TMS pain goes away. This happens most commonly with hay fever. I teach patients that all the conditions on the list serve the same purpose psychologically."

- "Experience with TMS, and these related conditions, suggests that there may be a common denominator, anxiety perhaps, that can bring on any of these disorders. In that case, some other emotion, anger for example, may be the primary one that may in turn induce anxiety, which then brings on the symptom."

Patients bring their medical history when consulting with a TMS physician. This information generally includes written physician reports, lab results and diagnostic imaging studies. After receiving a diagnosis of TMS, treatment begins.

The first step in treating TMS requires patient education. Physicians generally provide audio and written materials or recommend lectures. Education teaches the patient various aspects of the condition and reassures them that physical symptoms do not occur because of typical disease processes, physical injury or re-injury.

Another treatment modality physicians may use for treating TMS involves keeping a daily journal and writing about circumstances that might have created repressed emotional stress. David Schechter, M.D., recommends that when patients begin writing, they should consider whether they relate to certain key areas that often contribute to repressed feelings:

- Abuse, abandonment or neglect during childhood
- Conscientiousness or perfectionism related to acceptance
- Current life stressors
- Aging or mortality
- Situations wherein patients feel but repress negative emotions

After identifying a list of possible contributing factors, TMS physicians require that patients write an essay for each problem area. Longer essays allow patients to explore the issue in greater detail. Schechter developed a 30-day program called "The MindBody Workbook," which assists patients with documenting events that trigger negative emotions. The journal helps patients correlate the emotion with the physical symptoms of TMS. Over time, patients learn to use emotional expression rather than repression.

Part of TMS treatment also requires that patients live as if symptom-free. If physicians find no physical reason for chronic pain, Schechter advises that patients stop using conventional treatment methods for pain control. He believes these methods serve only to mentally reinforce a physical condition that does not exist. Patients must also resume normal physical activities when there is no physical evidence for pain.

Hypnosis

Nothing is more powerful than teaching your brain how to control pain and encourage healing. There are many forms of hypnosis and in some states only licensed psychologists can perform hypnosis on patients. The basic idea of hypnosis is to switch off the ideas in the mind that prevent one from achieving their goals. And thoughts like, "I am always in pain" and "Nothing ever helps" are negative mantras that keep one's mind and body locked in the pain cycle. The sooner these thoughts are released and replaced with positive ones, the faster the pain relief and recovery begin.

Look online and see what is available in your area, but be sure that "pain" is on the top of their list of specialties rather than hidden under a dozen other areas like smoking, anxiety, weight loss and others. Good hypnosis audio programs from reputable companies like The Hypnosis Network can also help you.

BAUD Therapy

The BAUD, or Bio Acoustical Utilization Device, is a new and powerful therapy tool. Invented by Dr. Frank Lawlis, a pioneer in the field of medical psychology, the BAUD is an FDA-cleared and registered device based on the latest discoveries of neuroscience.

The BAUD's patented technology utilizes specially designed sound frequencies and waveforms to quickly stimulate neural plasticity in a highly targeted way.

The BAUD is a neuromodulation device that works through neuroacoustic stimulation. It is unique because it doesn't require an external monitor. The client's sensations are used to monitor their neural response, and the client tunes the frequencies to achieve a desired result. In essence, the client's brain becomes the monitor. This provides a much more targeted and effective result and clients often see dramatic results in as little as one 20-minute session.

While we are still researching the exact mechanism of action of the BAUD, based on results so far, it seems to rapidly stimulate a parasympathetic response in very specific brain areas associated with the target problem. This brings neural function out of an aroused level, or sympathetic state, and produces often dramatic relief of the problem symptoms.

As therapists know, changing some negative feelings or compulsions is extremely difficult since the source is often unconscious. The brain areas negatively stimulated over many years can become stuck in a sympathetic, aroused response state. This energy then drives all sorts of unwanted urges or feelings or even physical symptoms. The client's attempts to change are difficult because they are fighting their own neural "programming."

The BAUD is effective in three main categories of problems: emotional issues, urges or impulses and physical symptoms like pain. This covers a wide variety of individual problems and we are continually discovering new applications for the BAUD.

We know from brain scans that merely shifting mental attention from one thing to another will "light up" different parts of the brain as neural activity increases. It is these active areas that the BAUD affects most strongly, creating a response that regulates, or normalizes the neural activity.

This means that any problem the client can focus on is potentially one the BAUD can improve. The BAUD provides relief in a way that most clients have never experienced. It gives them a powerful, pinpointed way to address the inner, neural source of their outer problem. They can focus on general anxiety or target any specific fear that limits them: heights, confined spaces, intimacy or even simply asking for a raise. They can reduce their appetite in general or eliminate only carb cravings.

And it doesn't take long to see results. A typical BAUD session may last from 15 to 20 minutes. Immediately after a session, many clients report feeling a profound improvement in issues that have plagued them for years, even a lifetime. While individual results vary, the relief they experience from just one session tends to be enduring, and the negative feelings diminish more with each subsequent session.

The BAUD is truly unique in the results it produces. Never before has this kind of relief been this fast and easy.

Learning to use and administer the BAUD is remarkably easy for therapists. It takes just minutes to learn the basic protocol. And most clients can learn to self-administer the BAUD as well. Some therapists have multiple BAUDs in the office to service several clients at once. Some have started BAUD rental programs.

With the BAUD you have a powerful tool with serious technology in a very simple and easy-to-use device. It gives you the power to help your clients in new ways. It gives your clients the power to turn problems "off" at their source.

Neurotherapists have reported that the BAUD has been a valuable addition to their traditional neurotherapy as a fast and effective intervention for addictions and traumatic emotional issues, as well as an effective way to quickly address pain issues and other physical symptoms.

Psychotherapists have found that the BAUD can help with a wide variety of psychological issues, and is especially helpful for PTSD and trauma-related problems, issues responsive to desensitization therapies like phobias, resolving past shame and guilt and even turning off those "hot buttons" in relationships.

Chapter Review

- Some people's acute and chronic pain is not related to a traumatic injury or arthritis; rather it is psychosomatic, meaning it is related to the way the mind and body interact
- If the physical body has been treated in every safe way imaginable but without improvement, looking at your thoughts and your emotions - a psychosomatic cause - may be the next logical step
- Thankfully, we have many safe, easy and powerful mind/body methods for eradicating chronic pain associated with negative thoughts and emotions
- I recommend Sedona Method, Emotional Freedom Technique (EFT), Tension Myositis Syndrome (TMS), as well as hypnosis, and BAUD Therapy

SECTION III:

The 30-Day Arthritis Relief Action Plan

CHAPTER 18

A Positive Attitude Supports a Successful Program

If you want to be healthy and happy instead of pained and sick, you have to readjust your attitude toward health. Healthy people are happy people. And shifting your attitude from "nothing helps" to "I can make better choices" is often the key step that offers optimal wellness and emotional fulfillment.

Health and happiness represent a frame of mind that influences our choices. In turn, making better lifestyle choices leads to wellness instead of chronic ill health.

Healthy Thought Processes

I know what you're thinking: "I didn't choose to be arthritic. It's not my choice to be in pain. I see specialists and practitioners to help my condition." I hear you. I know you are making your way as best you know how.

Healthy people seem to share certain characteristics. In fact, these characteristics are so prevalent among the healthy that those who share them could be considered a demographic. We are all familiar with demographics constructed around ethnicity, age, gender and income.

But did you know there is a demographic of the population that is concerned with a healthy lifestyle and green technology?

There is, and it's called LOHAS (Lifestyles of Health and Sustainability). LOHAS.com defines the group as, "A market segment focused on health and fitness, the environment, personal development, sustainable living, and social justice."

Not everyone who qualifies as part of the LOHAS demographic gains entrance by virtue of being healthy, pain-free and happy. However, it does seem that once people embrace this lifestyle, they become healthier and happier. Why? Because they have shifted their mindset, their perspective, from one of "nothing helps" and "I have to live with my illness" to "there are choices I can make to better myself."

Do you need to embrace LOHAS to be healthy and happy? No. Maybe worrying about green technology, carbon footprints, renewable resources and social justice is not your thing. But being healthy, pain-free, free of chronic illness and into wellness is something everybody wants.

I would like to share with you the characteristics (thoughts, actions and behaviors) most prevalent among those who are healthy. If you can begin embracing these, even one by one, you should see improvement, not only in your arthritis condition but also in your health overall and significant betterment of your quality of life.

Believe You Can Improve Your Wellness

While you may never be cured of your current health conditions, you can make vast progress in a short amount of time by having a better mindset and making better choices. A belief that your condition can improve is the motivational force necessary to feel better.

Own Your Present State of Health

Whether you see a medical doctor or alternative health practitioner, leaving your health in their hands does not significantly improve your condition. Owning your condition, taking responsibility for it and doing what you need to do to improve yourself are characteristics of healthy people. When you're mildly sick, do what you need to do to get well to prevent yourself from becoming seriously ill. Your health is yours, and no one cares as much as you do about improving it. Healthy people know this and take steps to promote wellness, not hinder it.

Know You Can Do It Yourself, with a Little Help

Roughly 80 percent of all conditions of pain, illness and disease are self-induced. That is to say, they are caused by the person suffering them. The problem is twofold: people don't know their conditions are self-induced and they don't know what they are doing to cause it. Consequently, they don't know what to do to change it. Healthy people know they cause their illness by their choices and behaviors and, therefore, can choose better and prevent them.

Make Choices and Stick To Them

One of the most difficult things people grapple with is sticking with a program for change. We choose to join the gym, but don't go. We make a series of appointments with the acupuncturist, but attend only three out of 10. Making strong wellness choices puts you on the path to wellness. Sticking to them and seeing them through keeps you on the path. Healthy people make healthy choices and stick with those choices, even when they are tired, under the weather or busy. And this characteristic is intertwined with the other three: belief, ownership and knowledge.

Keep an Open Mind

Health and wellness solutions come in all shapes and sizes. A few decades ago, chiropractic was seen as quackery, but today is a mainstream therapy. Ten years ago, acupuncture was still foreign to most Americans. While energy healing, meditation, polarity therapy, Reiki, herbal therapy and Prolozone therapy may seem strange or part of the fringe, healthy people keep an open mind about what can help their wellness. They may not understand something, but their exploratory nature and drive for a wellness lifestyle allow them to look into it, ask questions, interview a practitioner and/or experience an introductory session or class. Just because you are unfamiliar with a healing concept does not mean a solution is quackery. Keeping an open mind to new ideas and solutions can lead to an improved state of wellness.

Make Wellness Part of Your Lifestyle

The most important aspect of wellness is the fact that healthy people on the whole tend to make wellness a focal point of their lifestyle. If you carry a perspective of wellness with you when grocery shopping, you choose ingredients and foods that promote wellness, such as organic fruits and vegetables. When thinking of an afternoon activity during lunch break, the wellness-minded may choose a walk or quiet time rather than kvetching in the break room about co-workers that bother them. Rather than watching TV for two hours per night, the wellness lifestyle may find you doing yoga or QiGong or meditating or having a massage instead.

If your goal is to stop suffering by improving your overall health condition, then living a wellness lifestyle is a means to this end. There is an entire demographic of healthy and happy people doing it. You can do it, too. Do you need to fully embrace the LOHAS lifestyle and join the demographic to become well? No. But I'll bet that over time your wellness choices will impact your well-being and you will want to.

Chapter Review

- Health and happiness can overcome pain and sickness when you readjust your attitude toward a healthy frame of mind that influences your choices
- By making better lifestyle choices, you can find wellness instead of chronic ill health
- Model the thoughts, actions, and behaviors prevalent among those who are healthy
- Believe you can improve your wellness
- Own your present state of health
- Know you can do it yourself, with a little help
- Make choices and stick with them
- Keep an open mind
- Make wellness part of your lifestyle

CHAPTER 19

Setting SMART Wellness Goals for Success

Reaching your arthritis relief or wellness goals is no easy task. For many people, tackling such tasks, let alone setting goals to do so, can be daunting. Often times the perceived effort it will take to undertake the activities to achieve the goals, not to mention the time involved, seems more difficult than remaining in place. Thus, many people fall short of achieving their wellness goals, or end up doing nothing to achieve them.

That can all change, however, with a simple tool to help you develop and stay on track. The tool is a goal-setting concept called SMART. Each letter stands for the word that represents a component of an effective plan:

Specific
Measurable
Attainable
Realistic
Timely

Each of these five components is essential to both creating and achieving your wellness goals. Let's look at them in more detail.

Specific

The more specific you make your goals, the better chance you have of actualizing them. Specificity allows for understanding and measuring success along the other four areas of SMART. Without specificity, you will do more floating on the ocean than sailing on the seas. Driving in circles is never as fun or satisfying as directly reaching your destination. The more specific the details of the trip, the sooner you can reach the destination. And there can be more than one – a series of mini destinations – on the way to reaching the big destination over time. When working toward specificity, it is a good idea to begin by considering the five Ws: Why, What, Who, Where and When.

Why you want to change your state of health is the most important decision because it fuels your desire and sets your level of commitment to the program overall. Without knowing why, it is easy to do nothing.

What you want to accomplish is the next decision. Do you want to lose 20 pounds or increase your range of motion (or both)? The *what* of the matter is important for deciding on …

Who you need to involve. Wellness programs work best with a support structure in place. Who will you involve in the achievement of your goals? How about a workout neighbor, massage therapist, moral support from a loved one or a health care provider? Once these are all in place you will know …

Where all of this needs to happen. Do you require visits to an acupuncturist's office, or just a track to run around? What about the local yoga class or your living room?

When all this comes into play it is important for setting schedules and staying on track. People do better and reach their goals faster when they are in a routine. Knowing when to do what you need, is important to establish before you begin. Being specific is essential to knowing what goals you want to achieve and how to get there.

Measurable

Having measurable goals and a reliable metrics system are essential for achieving wellness goals. After all, without measuring progress how will you know if you've reached your goal, or mini-stops along the way? There are two parts to "measurable," the measured goal and the criteria for measuring it.

Let's say your goal is to lose 20 pounds in six months. Standing on a scale once per week offers the metric. Making a chart of progress at the end of each month, and measuring that against your hoped-for mini-monthly goals gives you the criteria for measurement. Other scales are also available, such as 1-10 subjective scales for things like pain, or hour scales for time (important for sleep measurements), or pH readings for your body's acidity level and so on.

The first step is to create a list of what you want to measure, and then how it can be measured. How much weight do you want to lose? How many miles do you want to run, or weight do you want to lift? How much of a decrease in pain do you want to feel each week, each month over what time? Being "specific" about these "measurements" will help you decide what is "attainable."

Attainable

If you can imagine it, you can achieve it. But the achieving is more likely to be attainable if the goals and vision are realistic enough to actually be attained. You must set an objective that you personally feel is obtainable and for which you are willing to put forth the effort. You can desire a long-off goal, but setting markers of achievement along the way will make it more attainable.

Many quit their wellness routines or drop their wellness lifestyles when they do not attain their desired goals in an immediate time frame as a result of the omission of mile markers. Listing small goals that will lead to larger goals is not only a successful way of attaining measurable results, but of building your self confidence, self belief and self image.

Realistic

In order for wellness goals to be attainable and measurable, they must be realistic for you. That is, they need to be something that you are physically, mentally and financially able to achieve. What identifies as realistic is a matter of personal relevance; you are the only one who can distinguish this.

Returning to an earlier example, if it is your goal to lose 20 pounds this must be realistic for you. If you are sufficiently overweight then losing 20 pounds makes healthy sense. But if you are not, then losing this much weight may be unrealistic and also unhealthy. Do you have the time and dedication to work toward achieving that goal? Do you have the financial and structural support necessary to allow it to happen? Moreover, being realistic means giving yourself several months to lose the weight, and not just a few weeks. Setting realistic time frames will go a long way to keeping you on track.

Timely

Timeliness is an important part of goal setting, especially when it comes to wellness. In what time frame are you trying to achieve your goals? How much time per day, week, and month are you planning on dedicating to the attainment of those goals? What time of day are you able to do this, to fit in with your overall life schedule? Being specific regarding your time is crucial. Just saying that you are "working on getting healthy" or on "the path of arthritis relief" is a statement that can lead to failure. Timeframes are important for goals to be measured in a meaningful way, not to mention realistic and attainable. Remember, be specific.

Once you have spent some time considering all of this and listing out the specifics of each of the five components, it's time to write out your SMART action statement. For example:

"I want to feel better and experience less pain because it makes me feel good and when I feel good I enjoy my life. I will lose 20 pounds and decrease my pain by 50 percent. To do this I will need the support of my family, a dietitian and a personal trainer, who is available on Wednesdays and Sundays. I will use a weigh scale and a pain index to chart my progress over the next six months, with mini goals set at the end of each month. I believe I can attain my goal because the time frame is realistic. I have a support system. I know what I need to do. I believe in myself and am dedicated to changing my own life for the better."

This statement is generic, but speaks to each of the five components of the SMART wellness goal-setting concept. Try it and see what a difference it can make in reaching your personal fitness, health and wellness goals. Let's now move on and discuss, specifically, the goals, objectives and strategies of the Arthritis Relief Action Plan.

Chapter Review

- Use the goal-setting concept called SMART to reach your arthritis relief goal
- **Specific** goals create better chances of actualizing them
- **Measurable** goals combined with reliable metrics are essential
- **Attainable** goals must also be **Realistic** enough to be achieved
- **Timeliness** is critical in setting goals for success
- The success of your Arthritis Relief Action Plan must be combined with SMART goals

CHAPTER 20

Program Goals, Objectives and Strategies

Here you are, at Chapter 20, where you finally get to read an overview of the Arthritis Relief Action Plan program. If you've read the book from the beginning, you will hopefully have a better understanding of arthritis. If you have not read the book from the beginning, please stop and do so. I cannot stress enough that for best results with this program you must understand the arthritis process, the components involved in slowing symptoms and why a portion of its damage can be reversed.

Without this understanding, it may be difficult to believe in the program, fully commit to doing it and seeing it through. If you have read everything from my Personal Message through Chapter 19, then you are well on your way to achieving program success and lasting relief from arthritis.

The power of the Arthritis Relief Action Plan program is based on its structure. I developed it with an integrated Mind/Body/Diet approach for a strong through-line (or scaffold) on which the various program segments are hung. We could also look at it like a tree: The roots are the information and knowledge upon which the program (tree) grows; the tree is the structure on which the program is based; and the branches are the actions and methods that will create positive change.

The Arthritis Relief Action Plan program is based on the following five "structures."

1. Gaining knowledge of arthritis
2. Having a strategy for success
3. Creating a personal vision statement
4. Setting long-term goals
5. Establishing short-term objectives

If you have read the book from the beginning, then the first structure – gaining information-based knowledge – is already complete. Let's take a look at our strategy for optimizing the success of the Arthritis Relief Action Plan.

The Strategy for Success

Without a strategy, not much can be accomplished. The most successful generals were victorious in battle partly because they had a successful strategy. Well, those who are at war with a debilitating health condition called arthritis need a strategy to overcome it. The strategy I developed for you is based on these principles:

1. Taking a DIY (Do It Yourself) approach is the only way to fully embrace the program, create wellness goals, change your environment, alter lifestyle choices to healthier options and create a better quality of life.

2. Seeking outside help as needed for specific things, including various hands-on therapies like bodywork, massage, FMS and BAUD therapy, acupuncture, fitness instruction and assisted stretching.

3. Using the SMART concept to help achieve success, by being realistic about my expectations and getting friends, family and coworkers onboard for support.

4. Embracing a natural and integrated mind/body/diet approach to change all aspects of myself that are needed to achieve positive results that last.

5. Creating personal long-term goals, short-term objectives, using various metrics to establish my current "set point" and track my progress moving forward.

6. Having everything ready to go before beginning the program, using the four days prior to the "first three days" to swap out bad foods and drinks for good ones; to have my first round of supplements and pain-relieving topical products on hand; to have appointments set for consultations or actual appointments with three wellness practitioners.

7. Being focused and ready to roll on day one because I have read this book, have the knowledge of the situation and belief in the program, and I am motivated!

Now that you can see there are well thought-out strategies in place, you should be more confident in the program and your ability to be successful in it. Let's turn that strategy into something more tangible, by fleshing out its pieces as they relate to you personally.

Create Your Personal Vision Statement

Creating your own personal Vision Statement is a great way to set a view of what you want to do and who you wish to become. How do you envision yourself now, the process of change and where you will be on the other end? To help you get started, here is my personal Vision Statement:

"My vision is to widen the reach of holistic wellness, bringing its message and methods to a broader audience through books, articles, webinars, personal health coaching and corporate wellness consulting."

Here is an example of a Vision Statement a person with arthritis going through our program might write.

"My vision is to become self-empowered, to take personal control of my thoughts, emotions and actions to fully embrace Dr. Wiley's self-directed arthritis program so that I may reduce my pain, increase my range of motion, change my life in positive ways that support wellness, and to finally regain control of my life and be happy."

Think about it for a moment and then try writing a statement of your own. Do this on a separate piece of paper or on your computer. When you have a succinct and empowering personal Vision Statement, write it below. You will refer back to this as you progress in the program.

My personal vision is to... ______________________

____

____

____

____

____

____

____

____

____

____

____

____

____

____

____

Set Your Long-Term Goals

Goal-setting is another powerful way to align yourself with your vision and the outcomes you desire. Without goals (general long-term desires) and objectives (specific short-term expectations), we would lack the focus necessary to move forward in positive and productive ways.

You can have more than one goal as long as they generically speak to the achievement or accomplishment of aspects of the program or your health and are based on implementing the methods outlined herein.

Goals are defined as *the purpose toward which an endeavor is directed, and the results achieved therefrom.* Here are examples of a few generic goals someone with arthritis might have.

Personal Goal - Example 1

My goal is to increase my range of motion so I can do more of the things I used to enjoy doing, like working with my hands, gardening and cooking.

Personal Goal - Example 2

My goal is to decrease my pain and reverse my condition over time so that I can feel better, resolve my stress and anxiety about my condition and enjoy a better quality of life.

Please take some time to write down several of your own goals on a separate piece of paper. Once you have them as you like, write them down in the space provided below. You will refer back to them as you go through the program.

Goal#1: ______________________________

____

____

____

Goal#2: ______________________________

____

____

____

____

Goal#3: ______________________________________

____

____

____

Establish Your Short-Term Objectives

Objectives are the specific targets you want to reach within the larger goal you set for yourself. Unlike goals, objectives are set for the short-term and are matched to metrics. In the case of our arthritis program, those metrics include weight, range of motion, pain, sleep, pH level and mental health.

Personal Objective - Example 1
I aim to lose 10 pounds in the first month, thereby reducing the compressive force on my arthritic hips and knees by 30 pounds, in an effort to reduce my overall pain level by 20 percent.

Personal Objective - Example 2
I aim to see a massage therapist, BAUD therapist and a personal trainer within the first month and attend all the required sessions.

Personal Objective - Example 3
I will follow the guidelines provided to change my sleeping environment and posture and to get an average of eight hours of reparative sleep every night by the first week of the program.

Please take some time to write down several of your own objectives on a separate piece of paper. Once you have them as you like, write them down in the space provided below. You will refer back to them as you go through the program.

Objective #1:____________________

Objective #2:____________________

Objective #3:____________________

Objective #4:____________________

Objective #5:____________________

Use Metrics to Assess Your "Set-Point"

Metrics are an important aspect of any program that has a certain success level as its goal. To overcome arthritis and reverse its damage, metrics are essential. They objectively quantify certain parts of the program and subjectively qualify how you are feeling along the way. I can't tell you how many times I treated patients for mixed pain syndrome (different kinds of pain in various places in the body), to have them tell me they don't feel any different. I would then take out their metrics chart, which they subjectively filled in, and show them that their headaches are down 45 percent, their sleep has improved by 60 percent and their inflammation is down by 70 percent. And of course they would say, "Yes, but my elbow still hurts!"

I joke, but in all seriousness you need a subjective assessment of several things to use the Arthritis Relief Program and be successful. Like your Vision Statement, goals and objectives, your personal metrics need to be written down. However, these also need to be updated every week for as long as you are on the program. This way, you will be able to chart everything each week and compare it with previous weeks on the program and with how you felt before beginning the program. This will let you know how you are doing in each of the essential aspects of what it takes to halt your arthritis from getting worse, to reduce your pain and to regenerate damaged tissues. Here are the areas to apply metrics to, and what you need to do.

Metric 1: Pain. Using Mosby's "Pain Rating Scale," please circle the number that most closely reflects how much pain you feel on a daily basis.

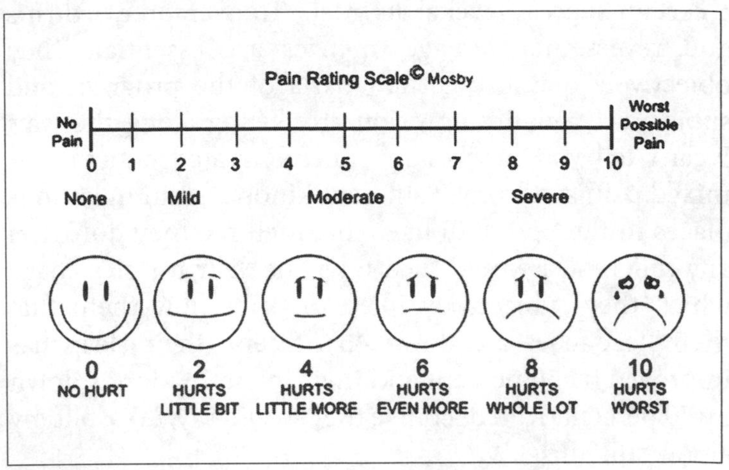

Metric 2. Emotional State. Using the "Emotions Scale," please consider your overall feelings about yourself in relation to your arthritis. You can circle all the feelings that you experience on a daily basis related to arthritis, but please only select one number for your baseline rating.

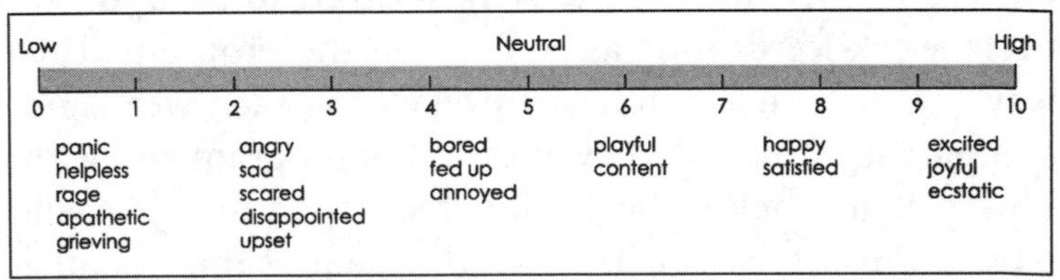

Metric 3. Stress. Measuring stress can be tricky because so many things are involved. There is both good and bad stress, and what is more important is how well one deals with their daily stress. If you are interested in taking a

comprehensive stress test, I recommend visiting http://freestresstest.org/ and take their 100 question online test. For our purposes here, please rate your stress level based on this question:

Thinking about the last month how stressed do you subjectively feel, when compared to times when you felt "life was good?"

Stress Feeling	Level
Not At All Stressed	0
Seldom Stressed	1 – 2
Sometimes Stressed	3 – 4
Frequently Stressed	5 – 6
Chronically Stressed	7 – 8
Nervous Breakdown*	9 – 10

*If you are feeling you may be on the verge of a nervous breakdown, please seek immediate medical attention or call a local therapist for help.

Metric 4. Sleep Quality. Getting good quality sleep is essential to feeling better as this is when the body repairs itself. Good quality sleep means sleeping in the correct posture, with duration of seven to eight hours per night, seven days per week, without disturbance, and awaking feeling refreshed. Given these qualifications, how would you rate your quality of sleep overall, over the past month? Circle one answer for each of the three qualifications, and then add your answers to get your total sleep quality score.

Sleep Quality	Poor = 1	Good = 2	Great = 3
Sleep Position	Stomach	Back	Side
Sleep Hours	4-6 hrs	6.5 7 hrs	7.5-8 hrs
Awaking Refreshed	Never	Sometimes	Always
Total Score = ____			

Metric 5. Body Mass Index (BMI). The Body Mass Index (BMI) measures your height to weight ratio. A BMI between 18.5-24.9 is within a healthy limit. Above or below is not so healthy. Please find the BMI number that connects your height and weight in the below "Body Mass Index Calculator."

BMI Chart

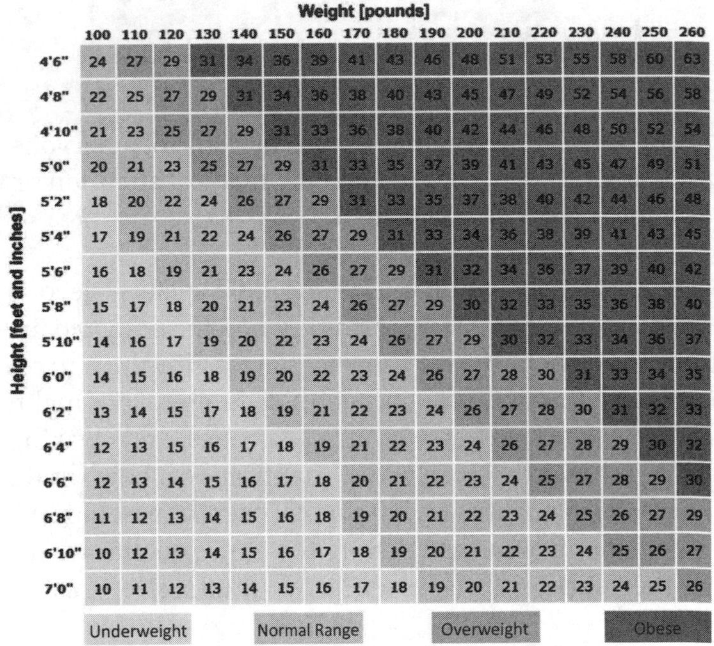

Weight [pounds]

Height [feet and inches]	100	110	120	130	140	150	160	170	180	190	200	210	220	230	240	250	260
4'6"	24	27	29	31	34	36	39	41	43	46	48	51	53	55	58	60	63
4'8"	22	25	27	29	31	34	36	38	40	43	45	47	49	52	54	56	58
4'10"	21	23	25	27	29	31	33	36	38	40	42	44	46	48	50	52	54
5'0"	20	21	23	25	27	29	31	33	35	37	39	41	43	45	47	49	51
5'2"	18	20	22	24	26	27	29	31	33	35	37	38	40	42	44	46	48
5'4"	17	19	21	22	24	26	27	29	31	33	34	36	38	39	41	43	45
5'6"	16	18	19	21	23	24	26	27	29	31	32	34	36	37	39	40	42
5'8"	15	17	18	20	21	23	24	26	27	29	30	32	33	35	36	38	40
5'10"	14	16	17	19	20	22	23	24	26	27	29	30	32	33	34	36	37
6'0"	14	15	16	18	19	20	22	23	24	26	27	28	30	31	33	34	35
6'2"	13	14	15	17	18	19	21	22	23	24	26	27	28	30	31	32	33
6'4"	12	13	15	16	17	18	19	21	22	23	24	26	27	28	29	30	32
6'6"	12	13	14	15	16	17	18	20	21	22	23	24	25	27	28	29	30
6'8"	11	12	13	14	15	16	18	19	20	21	22	23	24	25	26	27	29
6'10"	10	12	13	14	15	16	17	18	19	20	21	22	23	24	25	26	27
7'0"	10	11	12	13	14	15	16	17	18	19	20	21	22	23	24	25	26

Metric 6. pH Level. pH is a measure of the acid to alkaline level in your body. A pH of seven is neutral, and above eight is alkaline (healthy). The lower the number the more acidic (unhealthy) your body is. Please go to your local convenience story and purchase a pH testing strip or kit. You will use either your saliva or urine to get a reading. Then circle your number on the chart below.

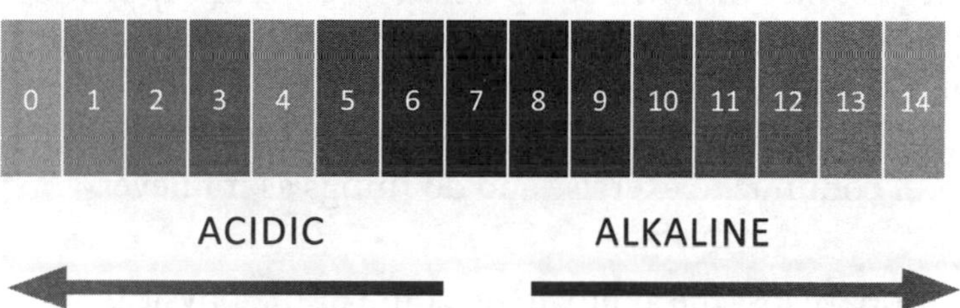

Metric 7. Range of Motion. To get a really good assessment of your actual range of motion (ROM) you will need to make an appointment with a physical therapist. You can also purchase a ROM measuring devise at http://www.quickmedical.com and take measurements, but this is often difficult on one's own. I suggest you take a moment and move each joint section and assess how you feel as you move front/back/sideways/in circles. Then select your current ROM state in the scale below.

My joints move as freely as they did before I got arthritis = 1 - 2

I have lost some ability to bend my joints in all directions = 3 - 4 - 5

My limited joint motion restrict many of the things I used to do = 6 - 7- 8

The Range of Motion (ROM) loss in my arthritis joints is severe = 9 - 10

Metric 8. Physical Activity. One of the worst things that people suffering arthritis deal with is their inability to do physical activity as they once did. But as you've learned, keeping active and moving the body and joints is essential to remain healthy, slow the arthritis progression and even reverse some of the damage. Thinking back on the past month, when compared to your "healthy prime," how subjectively do you feel you are able to exercise, walk and do physical activities?

I continue to exercise and do things as if I never had arthritis = 1 - 2

I have lost the ability to do some of the physical activities I enjoy = 3 - 4 - 5

Arthritis restricts many of the physical activities I used to do = 6 - 7- 8

Arthritis has made it nearly impossible to do any physical activity = 9 - 10

Your Arthritis Metrics Chart

Please fill in the below chart with your "Set-Point" metrics from the above lines. Together, these numbers will give you a snapshot of your condition and tell you how you feel now, prior to beginning the program. Then, after beginning the program and at the time allocated in the chart, please re-do your metrics and enter your new numbers into the chart. It would be great if you see steady progress over the course of a few weeks to a few months. However, it is not uncommon to feel a bit worse off at first, at least in some of the areas. This occurs because the body is being moved off its set point and is being led back toward balance (homeostasis). However, since getting arthritis, or even before then, it has found its new groove (a false sense of "balance") from being stuck in a symptomatic negative holding pattern.

YOUR ARTHRITIS METRICS							
	Set Point	7 Days	14 Days	21 Days	30 Days	60 Days	90 Days
Pain Level							
Emotional State							
Stress Level							
Sleep Quality							
Body Mass Index							
pH Measure							
Range of Motion							
Physical Activity							

Please know that while it is easy to think that having "bad scores" means there is no hope for you, in actuality the opposite is true. ***Those arthritis sufferers with the Highest Set Point have the greatest room for improvement*** and therefore have ***the best chance for marked improvement*** of their condition with this program.

Now that you have a clear idea of your "Set Point" prior to beginning the program, let's now continue on to Chapter 21 and learn about the best way to get through those tough First Three Days…

Chapter Review

- The power of the Arthritis Relief Action Plan is based on its uniquely integrated Mind/Body/Diet approach.
- The Arthritis Relief Action Plan is based on five "structures"
- Understanding the arthritis process, how to slow symptoms, and why some of the damage can be reversed is critical
- Your personal Vision Statement ensures you define what you want to accomplish and who you wish to become
- Goal-setting aligns your mind and body with your vision and the outcomes you desire
- Long-term goals and short-term expectations create the foundation to keep focus and move forward in positive and productive ways
- Metrics are essential to overcome and reverse arthritis, objectively quantifying certain parts of the program and subjectively qualifying your feelings through the journey

CHAPTER 21

Getting Started: The First Three Days

The first three days of anything requiring change are the hardest. This seems especially so when it comes to matters of health and wellness. The first three days of a new diet are a struggle, almost impossible it seems. The first three days of a new fitness program can seem unbearably painful and difficult. The first three sessions of a therapy (physical or psychological) seem to meet with the most resistance. But this doesn't have to be the case, and with an easier first three days, there are greater chances of success.

When people are not feeling well they seek the advice of a healthcare provider and hope for a fast cure, or at least some measurable help, for their acute symptoms. While scientific medicine has some very strong and effective symptomatic solutions, their effects do not often last or correct the cause of the imbalance. Unsatisfied with the short-term effects of bio-medicine, and their illness-causing side effects, many millions of people are turning to alternative therapies for gentler and more healthful solutions.

The problem is that most Americans want to have their cake and eat it too. In other words, they want to engage in alternative therapies like specific diets, herbal therapies, meditation and yoga sessions, mind-body modalities and various emotional therapies. But they want the solution to be powerful and immediate. Natural solutions take longer to help the body and thus by their nature are not toxic or harmful in the process. More importantly, natural wellness solutions often require that the person who is not well takes control and self-administer their "therapy." This is difficult for even the most sincere and holistic-minded person to do, as we have been raised to expect immediate results. Yet, fast results are not always the healthiest or longest lasting.

One of the main reasons people claim they have started and stopped diet plans and workout routines is because they could not "get into" the program fully because the first three days were "unbearable" for them. I have also crashed and burned within the first three days of my own health goals over the years, but was lucky to find a solution to the problem.

The solution I use with great success is to preempt those first three days with four pre-days. That is, I start to change my thoughts about what I will begin to do, and begin making changes to my habits and routines in small steps leading up to the first of the three days. Jumping into coldwater head first can be shocking and unbearable, causing you to jump right back out. However, dipping one toe and then another and then a leg and so on into the water, a little at a time, to prepare yourself physically, mentally and emotionally for the inevitable jump, makes the process much easier to handle and those first three days a delight to manage. Here are some things that I do during the four days leading up to day one of the "first three days" of my health changing activity.

Think From the End

Before beginning a new wellness activity, I spend some time thinking about the desired result and my reasons for wanting it. Whatever the reason, I consider it, meditate on it, think of all the wonderful things that will result from engaging in it. This gives me the emotional and mental "adjustment" into the need and desire of what I am about to do, so that when the program gets tough (and they all do at times), I won't quit. Being certain of why you want something, and having a burning desire to achieve it, makes success that much easier.

Get the Support of Others

One of the most common reasons people fall off their wellness programs is lack of support. Not only do humans tend to need someone to be accountable to but they also need to be part of a group. But often their social network is not on the same wellness path and can derail efforts by not respecting your changing needs and behaviors. I always tell my loved ones and co-workers before I begin a new program and ask them to ask me about my daily progress. Often people who need to change cannot do so on their own, but when a group of people in different places (work or home) ask them about it, they feel accountable and are more apt to do it. Additionally, if I am fasting or changing my diet I ask for support and buy-in from family and friends to understand and respect my changes and not be upset with me for not eating what they may be preparing for a meal.

Adjust Your "Set Point"

I refer to a "set point" as any metric on any topic. For instance, six hours sleep per night, three meals a day, 25 crunches; anything that can be measured in repetitions, hours, days, weight or other. For many people entering into a diet, their food set point can be measured in terms of meals per day, servings per meal, number of items or counts of calories or carbs or fats per meal, etc.

The concept here is to know where you need to be during the first three days of a new diet (for example). Then mitigate that stress and diet change jump-off point, but easing into it four days prior to the start. The same goes for stretching, exercise, meditation and so on. Begin readjusting your less-healthy "set point" so that the drastic change required of the new activity will not require as strong a shift and thus will be easier on the mind and body to handle and stick with it.

Change Your Environment

Another difficult piece that pulls many away from ultimate success is your living environment. If you are starting a diet, but have juices with high fructose corn syrup in the fridge, frozen pizza in the freezer, white bread on the counters and coffee calling your name, these items need to be removed. Out of sight, out of mind is a great saying that addresses the issue of psychological triggers. We often move on habit without thinking. Removing the unhealthy food from sight (or throwing it in the trash), putting the coffee pot into the closet, covering the TV (to help stay off the couch when we need to be out walking), and so on, helps reduce the subconscious triggers that arise from seeing things that are counterproductive to the new endeavor. If altering sleep is your issue, take the television and books out of your room prior to beginning a new sleep program. If engaging in therapies like EFT or EMDR or Sedona Method for changing past memories and emotional triggers, remove items and pictures and music from your surroundings that may trigger you and set you back in your success and therefore interfere with moving past the first three days and into the easier fourth day and beyond.

Be Specific on What the First Three Days Entail

One of the best things you can do to support your ability to manage and get through those first three days is to know exactly what you need to do and what you need to support that. For a cleanse or diet, that means having in your home and at your disposal from the first minute of day one, all the food or juice or supplements you will need to sail through those first three days and onward. Having the food and items at your fingertips from "go" makes the start and journey through the first days easier. Without all the thinking and shopping and scrounging to do what is required, the mental strain is lifted, the anxiety of not knowing what to do is eased, and only the emotional and physiological aspects are left to contend with. But, if you have been shifting the emotional set-point and other areas for the four days prior, as suggested, then those issues will be less of a strain and those first three days will be much easier, if not "painless."

The four pre-days leading up to the first three days of a new wellness program or diet or effort, are keys to helping enhance the process, make the transition on your mind, emotions and body easier, and help you adjust little by little so the deep-end dive that many do on day one will not drown them and their sincere efforts. With a four-day pre-set, the first three days can actually be a delight, and day one becomes day five.

Chapter Review

- The first three days will be the hardest
- Failures in diets, workouts, and other challenging programs happen when those first three days are too difficult or "unbearable"
- You can succeed in the first three days of the Arthritis Relief Action Plan, and it will not be as hard as most think
- Start changing your thoughts, make changes to habits and routines in small steps, and you'll be ready to succeed before you even start your first day
- Key strategies to prepare yourself for success involve thinking from the end, getting support, adjusting your "set point," changing your environment, specifying what the first three days will entail
- You can do it!

CHAPTER 22

The Arthritis Relief Action Plan

Now it is time to put into harmonious action the hundreds of pieces of information presented in this book into a wellness lifestyle that supports relief from arthritis and reversal of its symptoms. Below are charts outlining the seven major categories discussed in this book, and the solutions associated with each.

Implementing solutions from each of these categories forms the essence of the Arthritis Action Plan. The charts give you guidance into selecting best options within each category. You must, however, review the individual chapters to find the specific details of each solution and consider which resonate best with you.

1 - Dietary Solutions
Eat only pH neutral, alkalizing and anti-inflammatory foods
Drink enough pure water daily that your urine stream is clear
Drink 4 cups of green tea daily
Include mushrooms in two meals per day
Cook with a variety of thermogenic spices
Refer to Chapters 5, 6 & 10 for Details

2 - Supplementation Solutions
Take a daily supplement that helps reduce pain and inflammation
Take a daily supplement that helps support bone and joint health
Select a supplement that contains Proteolytic Enzymes
If applicable after a TCM diagnosis, take Chinese herbal formulas
Refer to Chapter 11 for Details

3 - Topical Product Solutions
Use only all-natural topical products
Select products that contain several active healing ingredients
Find and stick with products that give you fast, lasting relief
Don't be afraid of strange-sounding ingredient names
Refer to Chapter 12 for Details

4 - Ancient Exercise Solutions
Get up, get moving and remain active
Exercise for as long as you can without pain
Begin gently then increase in time and vigor
Begin with QiGong Standing Pole exercise
If you can do more, enroll in a Yoga or Tai Chi class
Mindful Walking is one of the best exercises!
Refer to Chapter 13 for Details

5 - Bodywork Therapy Solutions
Bodywork really helps with pain, inflammation, range of motion
Check local listings for bodywork practitioners
Experience many methods to find one that works for you
Don't be afraid of a little pain for long term gain!
Refer to Chapter 14 for details

6 - Energy Medicine Solutions
Remember, the body is electric and requires proper current
Pain, illness and disease are just low human vibrations
Check local listings for energy medicine practitioners
Experience many methods to find one that works for you
Some methods apply touch and some don't, but they still work!
Refer to Chapter 15 for Details

7 - Stress & Emotions Solutions
Remember: psychosomatic is a real connection!
Use the recommended "10 Stress Busters" daily
Do the "Relaxation Response" method every day
Meditate every day, at night or first thing in the morning
Get quality sleep in the correct posture
Don't be afraid to reach out to a therapist for assistance!
Refer to Chapters 16, 17 & 18 for Details

It is important that you include at least one thing from each category in your daily life. I highly recommend revamping your diet completely, and jumping right in with allocated times for "ancient exercises," stress reduction techniques, practitioner based bodywork and energy medicine therapies. I highly recommend setting appointments and times before Day 1, as discussed in Chapter 21, and having several different topical products and supplies of at least three supplements on hand.

Ideally, all of these seven categories should be approached at the same time. Yes, you can ease into them one per week or so, but the results will take longer. And please don't forget that assessing each area with metrics (Chapter 20) and updating those metrics weekly for the first 30 days is very important.

You might have noticed that the subtitle of the book is "The 30-Day Program..." and yet the Arthritis Metrics Chart has spaces for 90 days. The program for change and successful relief of symptoms is 30-days long. It takes about 30 days for most people to grasp all that needs to be done and to implement it, fold it into their daily lives. However, because everyone is different and requires a slightly different approach (e.g., different dietary changes, respond to different therapies, react better to different supplements and topical pain creams), adjustments need to be made for optimal outcomes. So it is a 30-day relief program that uses metrics to adjust the plan trajectory to garner best program synergy by the third month (90 days).

In other words, the first 30 days sets the tone, adjusts the attitude, reduces the stress, changes the diet, and welcomes new exercises and treatment modalities. Reduction in pain and inflammation and increased range of motion will be felt. But with a little patience and with some mindful attention to what is working best for you, you can adjust the "solutions" specifically for stronger results. You will know the results because of the metrics. By the third month you should be well on your way to once again finding homeostasis, a healthy and balanced body and life that is again full of joy.

The Arthritis Relief Action Plan works because it addresses the five essential components outlined in my "personal message" at the start of the book. These contain within them the elements for positive outcomes. It is my hope that the information in the book…

- Has educated you about the real causes and solutions of arthritis
- Can reduce the current level of symptoms you are experiencing
- Can halt or significantly reduce the worsening of your condition
- Can prevent symptoms from flaring to improve your quality of life
- Can regenerate healthy tissue to reverse the damage done

All you have to do to see positive results from the program is to:

- Take personal responsibility for your personal arthritic condition.
- Keep educating yourself by reading and rereading this book and online articles.
- Adjust your diet to one that is anti-inflammatory and immune building.
- Take supplements and apply topical products as needed to support symptomatic change.
- Practice ancient exercises and receive bodywork to help move blood and heal tissue.
- Receive some energy medicinal help to open energy pathways and energize.

- Practice stress relief methods and adopt better sleeping habits.
- Resolve your emotional issues that negatively impact your life .

I know this seems like a lot, but it really isn't. Actually, it's simply a refocus of your life. More simply put, it is about adopting a well-based lifestyle that is easy to follow once you are in the groove of it, so to speak. I wish you the best of luck and much success on your journal to a better, more joyous and pain-free life!

AFTERWORD

Break Down the Barriers to Success

How are you feeling now? Did you find something in the book that you may not have thought of or known about? I hope so. My goal has been to provide you with so much information, so many options, for arthritis relief and damage reversal, that you know there is hope for you and an improved condition. At this point, I know you are excited about the program and the positive outcomes that will follow.

I also know that despite best intentions, wishes and desires, you may stall, not proceed as directed, or even quit the program before best outcomes have shown. How do I know this? Because like you, I am human and I have come face-to-face with this in my life too. By *this*, I mean excuses. And excuses are like self-constructed barriers that erect in front of us and keep us from seeing our goal or even believing its achievable.

Whether you suffer stress or back pain, headaches or PMS, tendonitis or something else altogether, you have perhaps by now sought out alternative practices to relieve your suffering. Yes, the prescription meds helped a bit, for a while. But when they wore off, you had to take more … and more still. And now you are seeing an acupuncturist, a chiropractor, a massage therapist or some other holistic therapist and are finding that the requirements to do what is asked of you (even attending the frequent appointments), is just not quite fitting into your busy daily schedule.

Taking personal responsibility for your own health is difficult.

It requires dedication and patience.

Life can be tough.

Personal suffering is worse.

It seems we all, in our quest for health, well-being or simple pain relief, encounter the same set of barriers. These are things that seem either to be in our way or fall along our path as we traverse it toward a better quality of life. And while each person's barriers are of different shapes and sizes, the following three are by far the most common.

Barrier 1 – Time

Perhaps the most obvious barrier to achieving relief from arthritis is time. There is only so much of it in a day, a week, a month and a year. We can't add time, and when we finally do find a free moment it quickly gets eaten up by unsuspecting sources, like: work, house work, family obligations, events, projects, you name it. Something always seems to get in the way of doing our exercises, driving out of the way to purchase organic whole foods, eating balanced meals, getting a healthy amount of sleep, taking those supplements as directed, drinking enough water and exercising.

After a while, people start to think that going the "alternative" route to relief may be a bit overbearing. You have to visit the practitioner perhaps several days per week for several weeks or months. You have to take herbs or supplements – and handfuls of them several times per day. You have to do series of stretches or exercises between office visits ... and sometimes even on the same day. Who's got time for all that?

The main difference between mainstream medicine and alternative therapies is that the practitioners and products of alternative "medicine" are working toward healing you, not patching you up. Healing takes time and time is no true barrier to health.

I know you're busy. Perhaps, like me, you've got kids, a demanding job and a hectic family schedule. But if you need to exercise, you can prioritize at least 20 minutes, three days per week. Forget reruns of "30 Rock" or "Downton Abbey" – do your stretches instead. Better yet, why not do the exercises while watching your favorite sitcom or the evening news? Skip reading the morning paper and go for a walk instead. Avoid the take-out lunch and go to the farmer's market on the way home from work, then prepare a healthy lunch in advance.

There are always sets of minutes in a day that can be "constructed" into health minutes. You simply need to prioritize your day, your week – your life – and establish the time. If you don't and your ills become chronic or life threatening, what good is your time then?

Do yourself, your family and your loved-ones a favor and break down the time barrier. It doesn't exist; it's an illusion. Time is an abstract concept, but its utility can be physically modified on the fly. Only laziness and lack of creativity make time short. And we both know you're neither lazy nor uncreative.

Barrier 2 – Money

The second most common barrier to achieving perfect health is money. That is, having the financial means available to buy the best organic or free-range foods, receiving the best holistic treatments and taking only the highest quality herbs and supplements available. A personal trainer costs money. A weekly massage costs money. Acupuncture gets expensive. Herbs are cheap, but their protocols are long so their costs add up.

The main thing is to prioritize your wellness dollars. If you are spending X-amount on health each month, how can it be maximized? And if you are spending money on extra cable TV channels, expensive dinners and unnecessary clothing - then why not cut back on these and allocate the money for your health instead? Despite what you were told in the '80s, it's not how you look, it's how you feel that counts.

One of the best things you can do is to learn methods of reducing stress, stretches and exercises you can do by yourself at any time of day or night. This will allow you to reduce your massage frequency and you will derive greater benefit from the herbs and acupuncture you are receiving.

I recommend consulting your holistic practitioner to get a clear picture of how many visits over what length of time will be required of you. You also want to know what herbs or supplements you may need to take and over what period. With this information you will know ahead of time (no pun intended), how much money you will need to allocate for your natural therapy.

With this information, you can begin to budget your wellness dollars accordingly. I highly recommend you not begin a course of treatment until you have the means to attend every required visit and to purchase whatever additional things are needed along the way. There's no sense in wasting money on half a therapy. While you're pulling resources together, work on your sleep/wake cycle, stress relief and diet. With clarity of costs and allocation of money in place, there will no longer be a money barrier blocking your health.

Barrier 3 – Belief in the Outcome

The third most common barrier to health is you own level of belief in what it is you are doing (or receiving) and what the result of that will be. Are you on a diet? If so, do you believe it will do you good and deliver on the expected results? Are you receiving Tui-Na therapy or FSM Therapy? Do you think the sessions are helping, or will help if you follow them through their prescribed course of treatment?

My point is, many people who begin and then drop out of holistic therapies do so because they lose faith in the method of care they are receiving. This either happens because the practitioner has made unrealistic promises, or the patient was expecting different results than the ones gained. And most Americans want fast and easy results. Managing goals and expectations are key.

When working with alternative therapies of any kind, you must obtain a clear picture of what may and may not happen, and over what period. Managing your goals (e.g., "I want to be pain free by July 4") and your expectations (e.g., "At the very least, I expect to be gardening again in April"), you will be able to "stay the course" as the treatment progresses.

The best way to overcome the belief barrier is to discuss the therapeutic method at length with the practitioner who is offering the service. Ask for reading material. Ask for case studies. Talk to other patients. Put Google to work for you, too. By doing this, you will empower yourself with enough information to know that the program is either not the right one for you or that you can rightfully dedicate time, money and effort to it.

I understand that you may be at the end of your rope. You may have already spent huge sums of money, time and effort trying to get better, to be pain free, to lead the life you desire and so rightly deserve. But your life isn't over, and there is plenty of time left to truly live. All you have to do is redouble your courage, dig your heels in and:

1) **Make the Time**
2) **Allocate the Money**
3) **Believe in the Outcome**

By breaking down the barriers to health, nothing can block your path to the healthy pain-free life you so rightly deserve.

References

Chapter 1

Brodie, Richard. (2011). "Virus of the Mind: The New Science of the Meme." Hay House.

Eberhardt, Kerstin. (2004). "Experiences from a Prospective Early Rheumatoid Arthritis Study in Southern Sweden." *Journal of Rheumatology, 31* (69): 9-13. http://www.jrheum.com/subscribers/04/69/9.html

Chapter 4

Westrich, Geoffrey. (2011). "Top Myths About Arthritis." *The Queen's Courier.* http://queenscourier.com/2011/top-myths-about-arthritis-4227/

Chapter 6

CDCP (Center for Disease Control and Prevention). "Obesity Trends in Adults with Arthritis." http://www.cdc.gov/Features/dsStateArthritisObesity/

Cluett, Jonathan. (2009). "Joint Pain and Obesity." About.com.

Messier, SP, Gutekunst, DJ, Davis, C, and DeVita, P. (2005). "Weight Loss Reduces Knee-Joint Loads in Overweight and Obese Older Adults With Knee Osteoarthritis." *Arthritis & Rheumatism, 52*: 2026-2032.

Chapter 10

Cronin, JR. (2003). "Curcumin: Old spice is a new medicine." *Journal of Alternative & Complementary Therapies*, 34-38.

Egan, M.E., et al. (2004, April). "Curcumin, a Major Constituent of Turmeric, Corrects Cystic Fibrosis Defects." *Science (304)*: 600-602.

Haqqi, TM, Anthony, DD, Gupta, S, et al. (). "Prevention of collagen-induced arthritis in mice by a polyphenolic fraction from green tea." Proceedings of the National Academy of Sciences of the United States of America (PNAS), 96 (8): 4524–4529. http://www.pnas.org/content/96/8/4524.abstract

National Institutes of Health (2008). "MedlinePlus Herbs and Supplements: Turmeric (Curcuma longa Linn.) and Curcumin." US Department of Health and Human Services; Natural Standard Research Collaboration.

http://www.nlm.nih.gov/medlineplus/druginfo/natural/patient-turmeric.html

Sarker, SD, et. al. (2007). "Bioactivity of Turmeric," in *Turmeric: The genus Curcuma; Medicinal and aromatic plants–industrial profiles.* Boca Raton, FL: CRC Press.

Chapter 11

Arthritis Foundation. "Supplement Guide: Fish Oil." http://www.arthritistoday.org/arthritis-treatment/

natural-and-alternative-treatments/supplements-and-herbs/supplement-guide/fish-oil.php

Fitzhugh, DJ, Shan S, Dewhirst, MW, et. al. (2008). "Bromelain treatment decreases neutrophil migration to sites of inflammation." *Clinical Immunol*ogy, 128: 66-74.

Michael, H, Kinghorn, AD and JPhillipson, JD. (2004). *Fundamentals of Pharmacognosy and Phytotherapy*. Churchill Livingstone. p. 265.

Ugeskr Laeger 2005 Aug 15;167(33):3023-5. Find this abstract online at PubMed here: http://www.ncbi.nlm.nih.gov/pubmed/16109242

Wiley, MV. (2012). "The Essential Omega-3 Fatty Acids." Easy Health Options. http://easyhealthoptions.com/alternative-medicine/nutrition/the-essential-omega-3-fatty-acids/

Chapter 12

Braina, KR, Greena, DM, Dykesb, P.J., et al. (2006). "The Role of Menthol in Skin Penetration from Topical Formulations of Ibuprofen 5% in vivo." *Skin Pharmacol Physiol*ogy (19): 17-21.

Galeottia, N, Mannellia, LDC, Mazzantib, G, et al. (2002). "Menthol: A Natural Analgesic Compound." *Neuroscience Letters 322* (3): 145–148.

Hesslink, R, Armstrong, D, Nagendran, MV, et al. (2002). "Cetylated Fatty Acids Improve Knee Function in Patients with Osteoarthritis." *The Journal of Rheumatology,* 29 (8): 1708–12.

Leffingwell, JC and Shackelford, RE (1974). "Laevo-Menthol – Syntheses and Organoleptic Properties." *Cosmetics and Perfumery, 89* (6), 69-89.

Thomson Healthcare. (2007). "PDR for Herbal Medicines" (4th Edition), page 640.

Ting, Lillian. Publication on neurons, cellular reaction, medicinal qualities of menthol. *Science Creative Quarterly.*

Wiley, MV. (2013). "Try DMSO for Pain and Inflammation." Easy Health Options. http://easyhealthoptions.com/cancer/try-dmso-for-pain-and-inflammation/

Chapter 13

Wang, XJ and Moffett, JPC. (1994). "Traditional Chinese Therapeutic Exercises – Standing Pole." Foreign Language Press.

Chapter 14

Bensky, D and Barolet R. (1990). "Chinese Herbal Medicine: Formulas and Strategies." Eastland Press.

Chen, CH and O'Connor, J. (1981). "Acupuncture: A Comprehensive Text." Shanghai College of Traditional Chinese Medicine.

Guillaume, G and Chieu, M. (2002). "Rheumatology in Chinese Medicine" Eastland Press.

Purcell, Andrea. (nd). "Prolozone Therapy." http://www.portaltohealing.com/prolozone-therapy.html

Purcell, Andrea. (nd). What is Prolozone Theray?" http://portaltohealing.com/prolozone-therapy.html

Walton, AL (2011). "The effects of Quantum-Touch on Chronic Musculoskeletal Pain: A Pilot Study." *Energy Psychology*, 3 (2): 25-39.

Chapter 15

Carolyn McMakin, Carolyn. (2010). "Nonpharmacologic Treatment of Neuropathic Pain Using Frequency Specific Microcurrent." *The Pain Practitioner, 20* (3): 68-73.

http://www.frequencyspecific.com/papers/NeuropathicPain.pdf

Cheng, N, Van Hoof, H, Bockx, E, et al. (1982). "The Effect of Electric Currents on ATP Generation, Protein Synthesis and Membrane Transport in Rat Skin in Clinical Orthopedics." Clinical Orthopaedics and Related Research, 171: 264-272.

Hou, FX and Wiley, MV. (1999). "QiGong for Health and Well-Being." Journey Editions.

Chapter 16

Benson, H. and Klipper, MZ. (1975). "The Relaxation Response." Harper.

Wiley, MV. (2011). "10 Ways to Keep Stress from Killing You." http://www.drmarkwiley.com/blog/how-stress-is-killing-you%E2%80%A6-and-10-things-you-can-do-about-it/

Chapter 17

Dwoskin, Dale. (2003). "The Sedona Method: Your Key to Lasting Happiness, Success, Peace and Emotional Well-Being." Sedona Press.

Jacobs, Aaron. (2004). "Clinical Study: BAUD Assisted Neurotherapy." University of North Texas. http://www.mybaud.com/media_files/BAUDAssistedNeuroReport.pdf

Lawless, GF. (nd). "About the BAUD." http://www.baudtherapy.com/about_the_baud.html

Sarno, John. (2010). "Healing Back Pain: The Mind-Body Connection." Grand Central Life & Style.

APPENDIX

Chinese Medicine for Arthritis

Among the healing wonders of the world is the 5,000 year old tradition of Chinese medicine. Along with acupuncture, tui na massage and QiGong energy work is Chinese herbal medicine. This includes herbs made into healing teas, pills and topical pain relieving oils. For help in overcoming arthritis, the following traditional Chinese herbal products are recommended. It is best to see a licensed practitioner before choosing one, as their use is based on one's "pattern of imbalance" as opposed to symptom.

Du Huo Ji Sheng Wan

Du Huo Ji Sheng Wan is among the most powerful herbal patent formulas of Traditional Chinese Medicine (TCM). Its 14 combined herbs relieve the symptoms of rheumatoid arthritis (RA), rheumatism in general and sciatica through its action of "dispersing wind and dampness" (see Chapter 2 for descriptions of these). In modern terms, this herbal formula inhibits inflammation reactions and pain while improving the function of microphages to clear inflammatory tissue and increase blood circulation to reduce pain and swelling. Several studies have been carried out showing great improvement even when suffering arthritis for decades.

Kang Gu Zeng Sheng Pian

Another of the famous TCM patent herbal formulas, Kang Gu Zeng Sheng Pian, is also marketed under the English brand "Osteophyte." In my opinion it is an amazing formula used for a wide variety of joint and bone syndromes, such as osteoarthritis, rheumatoid arthritis, rheumatism and general joint pain, tendon pain, bone spurs, vertebral calcification following an injury, cervical spondylosis, subluxated or dislocated intervertebral discs, chronic cervical subluxation, spinal inflammation, osteoporosis, osteophytosis, Kashin-Beck disease, Heberden's nodes and heel spurs. It is found in Chinatowns and Asian markets as well as online.

Xiao Huo Lo Wan

This is my third recommended patent herbal formula from TCM. Xiao Huo Lo Wan is formulated from six herbs that are synergistic in their ability to alleviate numbness and decrease chronic pain in the hip, knee and ankle joints. It does this by invigorating the blood, resolving dampness that obstructs the channels of the body, dispels wind and dampness (see Chapter 2 for details on these terms). In Western scientific medical terms, Xiao Huo Lo Wan is shown to effectively treat arthritis (both RA and OA) and one-sided paralysis (hemoplegia).

White Flower Analgesic Balm

Popular in Asia, White Flower is an analgesic balm that works as a natural pain reliever for aching joints, headaches, sprains and backache. In addition to containing wintergreen, menthol and camphor, it also combines the essential oils derived from lavender, eucalyptus and peppermint, making it a potent aromatherapy agent. When applied to the body it has a soothing and calming effect on the nerves and emotions.

Red Flower Oil

Red Flower Oil is also widely used in Asia as a treatment for acute and chronic joint pain, muscle ache, sprains and bruising. In addition to wintergreen and camphor, Red Flower Oil blends several essential oils. These include clove, cinnamon and turpentine (a-pinene). Remember in Chapter 2 we discussed how Chinese medicine views arthritis as (in part) based on syndromes with odd names, like "wind-damp-heat," and so on? Well, Red Flower Oil is advocated for use in conditions that require dispelling of pathogenic wind, dispersing stasis (e.g., stagnations), activating the energy meridians of acupuncture and for relieving pain.

Po Sum On Oil

Po Sum On is a warming liniment with pain-relieving and anti-inflammatory effects. It is among the popular Asian topical products and is shown to be effective in treatment symptoms of joint pain, muscle aches, neuralgia, arthritis and sprains. Po Sum On is uniquely made from menthol plus the essential oils of peppermint, tea, dragon blood resin, cinnamon, scute and licorice.

Peppermint oil is both an analgesic (pain reliever) and antispasmodic (muscle relaxer). Dragon blood is a resin that aids in blood circulation and tissue regeneration. Cinnamon oil is a stimulant that aids blood circulation and reduces pain. Scute and licorice both help alleviate skin inflammation.

Tea oil comes mainly from the seeds of the tea plant; it has a light color and fragrance and a consistency like olive oil that gives this formulation its rich quality. Dragon's blood is the resin from Daemonorops draco, commonly used to promote blood circulation and tissue regeneration while relieving pain. Cinnamon oil is a warming stimulant to circulation and analgesic. Scute and licorice alleviate inflammation.

Wong Lop Kong Medicated Oil

Wong Lop Kong is one of my favorite medicated oils from Asia because it truly utilizes both essential oils and traditional Chinese herbal therapy. It contains camphor, safflower, peppermint, tea oil, frankincense gum resin and myrrh. Wong Lop Kong also contains dragon's blood resin, dang gui (agnelica), salvia root (danshen) and ligusticum (chuanxiong), making this topical product great for arthritis pain, rheumatism, bruises, blood clots and sprains.

About the Author

Mark Wiley, PhD, OMD, MSM is a doctor of both Oriental and alternative medicine, holds a masters in health care management, is a bestselling author, a martial art master and an international seminar instructor. No one does for wellness what he does.

Dr. Mark's interest in holistic and natural health practices began when he sought long-lasting relief from the debilitating migraines and chronic pain that plagued him for nearly three decades. In search of a cure, he traveled extensively throughout the United States, Europe, the Philippines, Malaysia, Singapore, Taiwan and Japan to conduct field research and master the world's holistic healing practices, from the oldest to the most modern.

Dr. Mark's passion for wellness has led him to become an innovator in the field of holistic health with the creation of the self-directed wellness model called, The Wiley Method. This method is unlike other healing systems that look at the individual symptoms and diseases and work toward managing them. Instead, it takes a system's view of health as being intimately tied to one's body, worldview and lifestyle choices. All symptoms of pain, illness and disease are considered within the context of the whole body, and the internal and external forces stressing its ability to maintain homeostasis – its optimally functioning baseline of health. In short, The Wiley Method provides a revolutionary way of providing recovery and then prevention of chronic pain, illness and disease.

In addition to his full-time health consulting practice, Dr. Mark is a prolific writer. He has written 500 articles and 12 books, most notably, "Natural Ways to Reverse and Prevent Hypertension" (Easy Health Options), "Outwitting Headaches" (Lyons Press), and "QiGong for Health and Well-Being" (Journey Editions). From 2003 to 2007, he was the Managing Director of Integrated Energy Medicine, LLC. He sits on the health advisory boards of several health and fitness institutes and associations, including The Healthy Back Institute and Easy Health Options, while focusing his attention on research, writing and helping people worldwide achieve healthy, balanced lives.